The Natural Apothecary

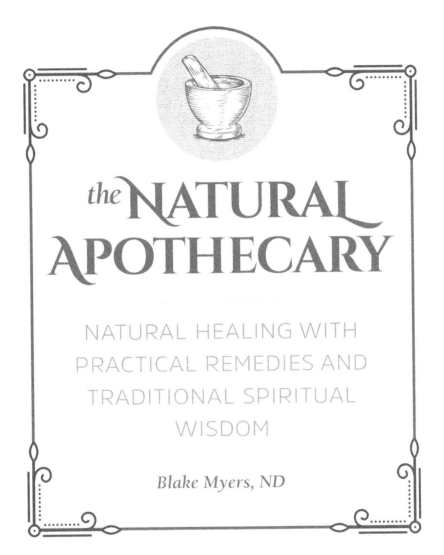

the NATURAL APOTHECARY

NATURAL HEALING WITH PRACTICAL REMEDIES AND TRADITIONAL SPIRITUAL WISDOM

Blake Myers, ND

ROCKRIDGE PRESS

To my beautiful son, Leonidas Starling;
to Jade, Cedar, Sage, Berkelly,
and all the littles in my life.
May you find new ways to
heal our Mother and carry forth her gifts
to the next generations.

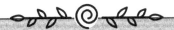

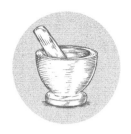

CONTENTS

PART TWO

REMEDIES FOR COMMON AILMENTS...31
REMEDIES GUIDANCE...32

INTRODUCTION

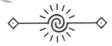

Growing up in a small town in southwest Iowa, I experienced the norms of the conventional medical system in the United States. In fact, that was my only exposure to medicine. It was all I knew and, I thought, all there was when it came to addressing health problems. At age 18, I enlisted as a medic in the US Army. Working in military clinics and the emergency room, I trained and worked in the standard American medical process. The emergency room was where I first decided I wanted to be a doctor. There were incredible physicians and nurses who truly inspired me.

As I went through my premed studies, however, I witnessed the detrimental effects of this system on my grandparents when dealing with aging and chronic illnesses. I reflected on my personal experiences as well as theirs and came to a conclusion that still holds true today. The conventional medical model is full of amazing scientific feats, and they're lifesaving in countless instances. However, when it comes to chronic illnesses—when the body and mind cannot get well on their own—there is a lack of solutions available. In fact, the majority of the tools utilized by conventional medicine are designed solely to suppress symptoms.

I'm interested in how the body heals. My mission is to resolve health problems by treating the cause and helping the healing mechanisms of the body work their magic. This is why I became a naturopathic doctor. I wrote this book to guide you through understanding natural medicine and how to use it to help yourself and others heal (and not just treat symptoms).

Information abounds on the Internet with "natural" treatments for anything from the common cold to cancer. The number of treatment options we can find is rarely the problem. What we run into is that most of us have a paradigm of modern conventional medical thought that influences how we use these options. This paradigm is ironically not one centered on healing. Herbs, nutrient supplements, etc. are just tools. The focus should be on the philosophy behind the decision of what to implement, when to implement, and the intentional use of these tools. In other words, we need to know what we're trying to accomplish and then pick the best tool for the job.

After digesting this material, you'll not only have a framework for maintaining wellness but also understand applicable treatment approaches for common chronic ailments. As you study the various conditions in this book, you'll start to see where there are overlaps, and you'll begin to be able to apply the information to other diseases and conditions as well.

When we blend good science and traditional wisdom, we have the opportunity to witness the magic of the healing process unfold. This is my hope for you. Enjoy this process—the experience, learning, and your personal healing journey.

HOW TO USE THIS BOOK

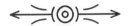

What you have in your hands is a condensed synthesis of current scientific understanding, traditional therapeutics, and my clinical experience, all imparted in a digestible manner. There are two parts to this book. In part one, we're getting the lay of the land of natural medicine. We'll cover some natural medicine history and the foundational components of health and gain insight into the framework you can use to create healing plans. Part two is dedicated to treatment considerations for specific conditions.

Although it can be tempting to go straight to a condition and start the therapeutics I've listed, you'll ultimately be better served by reading and reflecting on part one first. Healing from a chronic illness often looks different than what one might expect. There are ups and downs, setbacks, and big jumps forward. The first part of the book will help lay important foundations as well as explain how and when to reassess treatment and testing.

As you'll learn, good medicine and positive results in treating chronic illness is not a cookie-cutter approach. While it might seem that way when looking at a specific condition and the therapies I've listed, there is an art and individuality to what therapies to use and when. The desired results may occur the first time around, or it might take some experimenting with different combinations of therapies and different doses. Remember that *healing takes time*. Maintain a long-term vision, with a slow and steady mentality. If health and symptoms improve 10 percent in a month, celebrate it. If that trajectory is maintained, imagine where you'll be in a year.

Anyone suffering from chronic health problems—and the family, friends, and caregivers of those with chronic conditions—will surely benefit from the information in this book. Those who are relatively healthy will find the information here beneficial for preserving wellness and will also gain natural options for common conditions that may arise. This book will also benefit practitioners who aren't trained in natural medicine but want to incorporate safe and effective therapeutics in their practice. This book can serve as an easy desktop guide for any clinician to have handy for quick reference for nutrient and herbal options they can confidently prescribe to their patients for common conditions.

DISCLAIMER: *For nonpractitioners: The treatment information contained in this book is not meant to serve as direct medical advice, but rather, as an informational and educational resource. No action should be taken based solely on the information in this book. Although the natural therapies listed are generally safe adult doses, readers should always consult with a medical professional regarding their health. Doing so ensures the decisions you make are the best for your individual case as well as safe with the other medications or supplements you may be taking. Never attempt to self-diagnose a condition. Diagnosis is best left for medical providers who understand the testing, diagnostic criteria, and any different diagnoses that need to be ruled out. Readers who fail to consult appropriate health authorities do so at their own risk of injury or harm. The author and publisher bear no responsibility for errors or omissions.*

For practitioners: The doses listed for herbs and nutrients are generally safe adult doses. Doses need to be adjusted appropriately for children. Although every effort has been made to avoid errors, it's always recommended to consult peer-reviewed research and professional monographs whenever possible before utilizing treatments with patients. The information here is to help you have a framework to help treat patients with chronic illness effectively and to provide natural medicine options for your consideration. Always choose what is most appropriate for the case in front of you.

PART ONE

GETTING *the* MOST *from* NATURAL MEDICINE

The pursuit of understanding health and healing has existed for ages. In every part of the world, there are rich healing traditions. Natural medicine users today carry the torch of this ancestral wisdom. Those of us steeped in the world of natural healing owe our origins to those past, keen observers of nature and the human experience. To realize the full potential of natural medicine, we must first maintain these traditional roots. Then we can build upon them with our ever-deepening understanding of the science behind the natural world.

Before we discuss holistic therapies, I want to introduce you to some fundamental concepts. Chapter 1 will give you a basic understanding of the larger systems of medicine found throughout the world, their philosophies, and their approaches to treatment. The other important introductory component we will cover is the definition of the term "natural medicine." It can sometimes be confusing to know what it does and doesn't include. We'll explore this concept.

By learning a brief history of natural medicine and how to define it, we will begin our journey toward addressing the root causes of common illnesses with natural therapies.

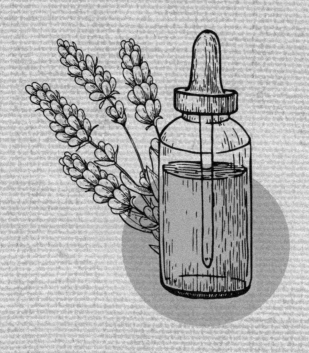

CHAPTER 1
OVERVIEW and HISTORY

"Natural medicine" is somewhat of an umbrella phrase. It's a broad term that encompasses many different healing systems and philosophies. Opinions may vary in regard to exactly what is included or excluded in the definition, but there are some typical overlaps and generally accepted ideas.

Most commonly, natural medicine means the use of substances found in the natural world to facilitate healing, or at the very least to treat symptoms. Natural substances could be plants, animals, minerals, water, air, sound, vitamins, and so on. This also includes therapies like massage, craniosacral, and acupuncture. Effective natural healing modalities are based on natural principles and tend to be rooted in basic sciences. In my view, natural medicine is a way of working *with* a natural system, in our case the human organism, versus forcing an action on the system. This distinction means that when using natural medicine approaches, we are utilizing the inherent healing capacities of the body in order to see results.

"Eastern" and "Western" are terms commonly used in regard to medicine. Oftentimes people perceive Western medicine as our current, conventional healthcare system. However, the more traditional medicines (which are not necessarily native medicine) of the West involve therapies such as hydrotherapy and Western herbalism. Examples of Eastern traditional medicine are Ayurveda and East Asian Medicine, sometimes also called Oriental Medicine.

Root Cause Healing

The primary question we need to consider in healing is, "What is the *root cause*?"—the root being the deepest or most foundational cause. The answer always is that it depends, both on how deep you look and on your perspective. Some healing traditions may see life force aberration as the root cause. Others may view differing levels of causation. With chronic illness, there are usually a variety of causative and contributing factors. Let's look at a real-world example.

A 65-year-old man goes to his primary care doctor because he has nerve pain in his feet (i.e., neuropathy). The doctor thinks, *His foot pain is caused by his nerves. If I give him medication to calm the nerves and slow down conduction, his foot pain should improve.* The doctor prescribes Gabapentin and it helps some, but the patient goes to see a naturopathic doctor (ND), as the neuropathy isn't yet resolved. The naturopath looks at lab work and discovers the patient is B_{12} deficient. The doctor provides the patient with B_{12} shots and, in turn, resolves the neuropathy.

But why was the patient B_{12} deficient in the first place? Dig deeper and we'll find this patient doesn't have enough stomach acid, which is required for B_{12} absorption. Why doesn't he have enough stomach acid? Aging? Maybe. Look further and we find that he started having other digestive problems a year ago. What life events took place a year ago? The death of his partner, which caused him to eat less and develop digestive problems. We can, and arguably should, treat the different levels of causation that we find along the way. Herbs that support stomach acid production and digestion in addition to B_{12} injections makes really good sense. However, if we're trying to treat the root cause, we will help this person most completely by supporting him with the grieving process and rediscovering his joy and purpose in life again.

Keep in mind that the life force of this individual is ultimately affected here also. What's important to understand is that you can work directly with the life force, or take an approach like in this example, and the life force will restore balance.

Let's look at some examples of traditional medical systems and their approaches to root cause treatment.

East Asian Medicine

East Asian Medicine (EAM) encompasses the traditional medicine practices of the large geographic regions of China, Japan, Korea, and the surrounding areas. Many of these medical practices have been around for thousands of years. Traditional Chinese Medicine (TCM) is a commonly accessible form of EAM in many parts of the world, that includes a large and growing evidence base to support its effectiveness for treating a wide range of diseases and managing pain. By working with the natural patterning and processes of the body and our environment, Chinese medicine aims to eliminate the root cause of disease, not just simply mask symptoms.

In Chinese medicine, qi, sometimes described as life energy, and the equal and opposing natures of yin and yang are the foundations to facilitate healing. Yin and yang need to remain in a healthy balance in order to maintain optimal health. Yang is the quality of heat and excess and is external in nature. Yin has the opposite qualities; cold, deficient, and internal. Practitioners use therapies, primarily acupuncture, herbal medicine, and physical medicine, to restore and maintain this homeostasis. This is achieved by promoting circulation of qi, blood, and body fluids, and restoring the proper relationship between yin and yang.

This process of promoting the circulation of qi, blood, and body fluids, is an excellent example of what is meant when I describe facilitating healing in this book. The practitioner supports these natural processes and the result is what the body does inherently—heal.

Ayurveda

Ayurvedic medicine originated in India many thousands of years ago. Literally translated, Ayurveda means life science, or knowledge—it's the science of life. If our goal is to optimize and preserve life, understanding the science of life may not be a bad place to start. According to Deepak Chopra at the Chopra Institute, there are two primary principles in Ayurveda.

1. The mind and the body are inextricably connected.
2. Nothing has more power to heal and transform the body than the mind.

Similar to qi, prana is the life force recognized in Ayurvedic medicine. Prana must be maintained in order for life and health to flourish. Prana can be worked with using pranayama, a yoga practice that focuses on breathing. This consists of various techniques used to control and move the breath, and subsequently the prana, through the body.

Another foundational concept in Ayurveda is that of the doshas. These are like "constitutions," or ways in which an individual experiences and adapts to the world. There are three types of doshas: vata, pitta, and kapha. An individual can exhibit the primary characteristics of one of these doshas or an overlap of several. Based on a person's dosha makeup, certain foods, herbs, and other treatments are used that are specific to them.

Western Herbalism

It's fair to say the use of herbs and plants as medicine is common throughout most, if not all, cultures. Western herbalism (WH) is a term meant to differentiate traditional herbal medicine of Anglo-American origin from herbal medicine practices of other large systems, such as EAM.

Other names you may also hear that are synonymous with WH are herbalism, herbal or botanical medicine, and possibly medical herbalism or phytotherapy. WH is commonly practiced in countries like the United States, Australia, New Zealand, the United Kingdom, and much of Western Europe.

Currently, WH is a mix of traditional uses combined with more modern scientific knowledge. There are constitutional approaches used by some in WH, but the most common practice is using herbs to support various body systems (i.e., cardiovascular, digestive, etc.). Western herbalists frequently describe plants by their actions. For example, the herb Lemon Balm (*Melissa officinalis*) has actions of nervine (calming), carminative (prevents gas/digestive support), and antiviral support. So, when I see someone who is typically amped up before bed and has trouble falling asleep, nervine is an action that warrants the use of Lemon Balm. Likewise, if they have a cold sore, I might use it for its antiviral action.

Shamanism and Energy Healing

Many cultures have come to understand the root cause of illness to be spiritual or energetic in nature.

Shamanism may be the oldest human tradition related to healing. Shamans are individuals who possess the ability to directly communicate and work in the spirit realm. These people can communicate with all spirits—plant, animal, human, stone, etc. A shaman can perform essential healing work such as retrieving lost or fractured pieces of a person's spirit, for example. In Western cultures, it's increasingly common to encounter those who describe themselves as shamanic practitioners. Shamanic practitioners have been trained in various techniques and ceremonies, like how to journey into the spirit realm or a cord-cutting ceremony. Traditionally, however, a shaman is born into this role in a community.

Energy medicine takes many forms depending on the practitioner, their experience, and training. Sound, magnetism, and light are all examples of energies. In addition, there are many subtle energies with which one can work to facilitate healing. Adding to the complexity of energy medicine, there are numerous ways through which to perceive energy. Some people may see energy fields. Others may feel them with their hands; others may sense them on a more intuitive level. Shifting energy into an area where it's absent, or moving stagnant energy out of an area, are two examples of how to support healing in this way.

Naturopathic Medicine

PRINCIPLES OF NATUROPATHIC MEDICINE

1. First, do no harm (*Primum non nocere*)
2. The healing power of nature, or vital force (*Vis medicatrix naturae*)
3. Identify and treat the cause (*Tolle causam*)
4. Treat the whole person (*Tolle totum*)
5. Doctor as teacher (*Docere*)
6. Prevention (*Praevenic*)

NOTE: *When I talk about NDs or naturopaths in this book, I always mean practitioners who went to a four-year, post-graduate naturopathic medical school. Due to the current regulatory nature in the United States, there are many people who can call themselves naturopaths and even naturopathic "doctors" who are anything but doctors. They attended an online certificate program. Please make sure your ND attended a university accredited by the Council on Naturopathic Medical Education (CNME).*

Naturopathic medicine is eclectic and broad, both in the therapies used as well as the styles of practice of NDs. Naturopathic medicine was originally a broad mix of therapeutic approaches, such as Western herbalism, hydrotherapy, diet, lifestyle, counseling, movement, physical/body manipulative therapies, and homeopathy. While naturopathy has largely retained its therapeutic origins, much more has been added as scientific advances have come along. Depending on the therapies a particular ND gravitates toward, what peer-reviewed scientific research shows is effective, the scope of practice for a particular state, and what the clinician has experience with, you'll now find NDs who also use therapies like biofeedback, hyperbaric oxygen therapy, and IVs.

NDs focus on treatment approaches that will be sustainable, realistic for your lifestyle, as well as effective and well tolerated. Aside from root causes of illness, the foundations of health will also be addressed. These are the foundational components required for life to exist in a healthy way. They include: the foods we eat or don't eat; what and how much we drink; our stress levels and how we manage stress; sleep; relationship health; movement; rest; and spiritual/religious/purpose orientation.

This list isn't exhaustive but conveys the idea. Naturopaths typically work to help improve and optimize these foundations of health, while also treating causative factors of illness. Sometimes these foundations are the cause.

NOTE: *To clarify a common point of confusion, homeopathy is a system of medicine all its own. Some NDs are homeopaths, and some aren't. Likewise, many homeopaths aren't NDs.*

Naturopathy vs. Allopathy

Allopathic (conventional) medicine is, at its core, a reductionist and mechanistic model. It uses the scientific method to try and reach its goals. The basic premise is, if we can just see a little bit smaller—if we can just see this gene, that receptor, this enzyme, etc., then we can develop a treatment (usually a drug) to affect it in some way. This approach has been exceedingly valuable in many acute and emergency situations. If we are having a stroke, there are drugs to break the clots blocking blood flow. If our body is overrun with "bad" bacteria, antibiotics can be amazing and lifesaving. Where the conventional system falls short is in the treatment of chronic illnesses. That's because healing chronic illnesses versus managing them often requires various lenses and more than the purely reductionist view.

Chronic illness can be complex. It's ultimately better addressed using a combination of reductionist scientific analysis with constitutional and body systems support. It needs a holistic perspective. Using only allopathic thinking often leads to simply treating symptoms. Symptoms to a holistic practitioner aren't the problem to be fixed; they're the road map to the healing process. If healing is our goal and it's taking place, symptoms will resolve on their own.

NDs go through a rigorous basic science education. We learn diagnosis, in-depth normal and abnormal physiology of all the body systems, comprehensive anatomy, and biochemistry in the same fashion one would expect for any competent clinician. This results in the same diagnostic and scientific understanding of medical conditions as other medical professionals. While that similarity is present, **what is different is the therapeutics NDs have available and the way we're thinking about the cause of disease and *how to facilitate healing*.**

Activating the Inner Healer

The last time you got a cut on your finger, what did you do to make it heal? Nothing, right? You may have used an antibacterial ointment on the cut and kept it covered, but that's likely all. That's because there are inborn mechanisms in your body to heal from damage that you don't have to think about or try to make happen. No more than you have to think about making your heart beat.

Sometimes though, something gets in the way of healing. Perhaps there is a traumatic event and the healing process gets interrupted or impeded; or maybe there is minor, long-term damage that slowly builds up over time, like from unmanaged hyperglycemia (high blood sugar).

In these cases where illness becomes chronic, the body, mind, and/or emotions, get stuck in a cycle. We need to break that cycle, and it can be a lot easier than one might think. Often, to experience a different outcome, the solution is to merely try something different than the day-to-day status quo. Little changes go a long way. Start now, wherever you're at. Small changes, in the long term, bring big benefit.

Whatever your individual case may be, trust that your body has an innate capacity to heal. Take comfort in this. Even if you feel like you've tried everything, know that there are always more options and solutions available.

Here is a three-step framework to help yourself and others heal.

1. **OBSTACLES.** What are the obstacles to healing? Is there anything keeping you from feeling well? Remove these obstacles if at all possible. If you remove any obstacles, improvement will start to happen.
2. **FOUNDATIONS.** Of the foundations mentioned previously, which ones do you think deserve attention? Which ones do you think play the biggest role in your health? What do you have control over to actually affect?
3. **JUST ONE THING.** If you could change just one thing to help yourself feel better, what would it be? All you need is one. You don't have to have all the answers today, just a place to start.

The Take-Home

If you can grasp one concept regarding healing, make it this: healing is natural! Only the human organism, in its inherent capacity, has the capability to heal. No medication, supplement, herb, or procedure can *make* the body heal. What we *can* do is *facilitate healing* and *remove obstacles*. Please take a moment here and reflect on this concept. It's a simple, foundational concept, yet profound in its effect. In my experience, this is a universal truth that many medical practitioners don't fully embrace. If you appreciate this reality and keep it as your guiding beacon along the way, you'll be ahead of many in the medical community. If we are able to understand what health is, recognize how healing happens, and what stimulates it to happen, then we can begin to help ourselves and others heal. Remember, the practitioner doesn't do the healing; the patient does.

Remember, the practitioner
doesn't do the healing, the patient does.

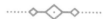

As you begin to practice natural medicine, you'll find it's inherently empowering due to its accessibility and efficacy. The vast array of powerful tools at our disposal in the natural world is our shared collective medicine. Its conservation is, therefore, also our duty. Our use of the natural apothecary requires us to be stewards of the planet, in order to preserve and protect our valuable medicinal resources for both ourselves and future generations.

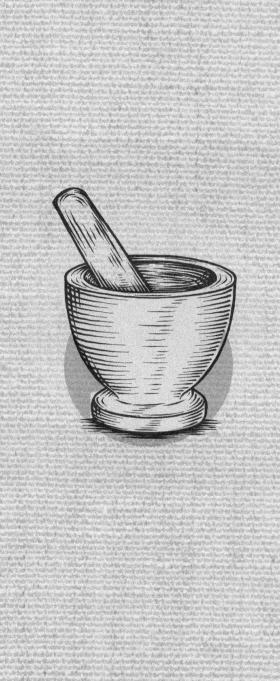

CHAPTER 2

THE PILLARS *of* GOOD HEALTH

Whether you are relatively healthy and want to maintain that health or have chronic symptoms and want to overcome them, there are some basic tenets to follow. These are the foundations, such as movement, rest, food, etc. mentioned in chapter 1 (page 3). These foundations are not just helpful; they're conditions for health. They are requirements for us all, to not only feel well, but also for our physiology and natural healing mechanisms to function properly. If you only focus on improving and optimizing these things, you'll have set the stage for wellness. Conversely, if these things are ignored, health and healing are less likely to be realized. You can't grow a vital plant from one that's living in poor soil. The same is true for us. This chapter is about tending to our soil.

Mindset

The mind-body connection is more than a communication between two separate parts. It is more like saltwater: conceptually separable, but when in solution, more like one entity. When we have a thought or emotion, our physiology changes in tandem. Likewise, when we have a bodily experience, our mental and emotional experience shifts with it. We can change our mental and emotional reality, perhaps something like anxiety, by changing our body. The opposite is also true. We can shift our bodily experience and physiology in the moment, and for the long term, by changing our mental and emotional spheres. By consciously modifying our mindset, we also shift our behavior choices, like what we eat, how much we exercise, and how we spend our time.

Viewing a healthy mindset through a lens of what facilitates happiness can be a useful model. Happiness is comprised of several factors, such as feelings of joy and pleasure, a sense of meaning and purpose in life, and life satisfaction. Although the relationships are not all clear, happiness is correlated with a decrease in all-cause mortality (risk of dying from anything). Meaning, facilitating happiness is good for us on many, if not all, levels. Here are some ways to increase happiness, shift perspective, and bring inner calm into your life.

Show Gratitude

Reminding yourself daily of what you are grateful for affects overall perspective and can help teach your brain to see both sides of life (i.e., the negative and positive). Write down three things you are grateful for each day in a journal. Try writing different things each time. For a challenge, think of a frustrating or negative experience and write something you're grateful for from that experience. For example, perhaps someone was aggressive in traffic and upon reflection, you are grateful for the ability to react quickly and safely in the moment. That shows gratitude for what you can control, instead of focusing solely on the negative interaction. Spend the next month writing down three things you're grateful for each day and see how you feel.

Meditate

Spend 15 minutes a day sitting in a calm, quiet space. Gently close your eyes and notice your body. Notice your breath. Let the outside world go and sit with yourself. Know there is no right or wrong way to meditate; there's no such thing as being "good" or "bad" at meditation. It's simply a practice in being present, which on some days is easier to accomplish than others. As your mind wanders (and it always will), work on gently and compassionately bringing your attention back to your breath or any other place in your body you would like to focus on. Taking this time, and the repeated returning to self, is the practice and the medicine of meditation.

Create Rituals

Our bodies and brains respond very well to routine and ritual. Consider what rituals you already have in your life. Taking teatime daily or watching a favorite weekly TV show, are examples of rituals. Where we have rituals in our lives, we will inherently find the things to which we give meaning. Begin the ritual of making *you* time. After waking up in the morning is a great time for a ritual. This is when I pray, give my gratitude, and set my intentions for the kind of day I want to have. I do this all while waiting for the water to boil to make coffee (another ritual). Take time daily for your meditation, gratitude, and praying, if that's in your belief system. If praying isn't your thing, practice journaling, or verbalizing, what you wish to see manifest for your day, month, or even year. Bringing your thoughts and desires into physical form in this way creates the space for them to manifest into reality.

Be Compassionate

Compassion usually feels easy when the situation is low stress or we're not emotionally triggered, such as feeling angry or afraid. I encourage you to practice awareness of your emotions and explore what it looks like to have compassion for others who have harmed you or upset you in some way. This is a tall task, no doubt, but essential for our personal as well as societal evolution, into a space of increased love, acceptance, and connection.

Feed Your Spirit

Simply put, do things that make you feel vital, excited, and alive. Do one thing daily, if possible, and at least a couple of times a week. What gives you an exuberant feeling in your body and mind? Is it outdoor activity, like mountain biking, fishing, or surfing? Experimenting with a new food recipe? Art or music? Whatever it is, when you get that exuberant feeling, it's because your spirit is resonating with the activity. Feeding this will benefit you on all levels, as your spirit responds to living its passions.

Lifestyle

Lifestyle may technically be a noun, but I suggest we all make it a verb. Style, according to the Merriam-Webster Dictionary, can mean to "design, make, or arrange." Life-design . . . now that feels liberating and exciting! We have a choice over so much in our lives that deeply affects our well-being. Here are two deeply impactful lifestyle ingredients you have control over. Use this guidance as a starting point to design your life for better health.

Sleep

Sleep is not only important for health, but also required for survival. You can't live without sleep any more than you can live without food or water. Some of the areas commonly affected by sleep are memory, cognition, mood, and resilience to stress. Inflammation also increases with decreased sleep. The scientific consensus is that seven to eight hours a night of uninterrupted sleep is the optimal amount for most people.

There's always more to do in a day, but make sleep a priority. Start practicing a bedtime ritual. At least 30 minutes before bedtime, turn off screens and slow down. Find something that relaxes you. Perhaps making of cup of calming tea, like Lemon Balm or Skullcap, or listening to some soothing music. Whatever you decide, begin this ritual around the same time each night. Be consistent. Keep your sleeping environment cool and free of screens. Make where you sleep a sanctuary for restoration.

NOTE: *Insomnia is a very common condition and specific advice regarding this will be given in part 2.*

Movement

Movement is what the human body was designed to do. JustStand.org is an organization with the mission to combat the negative effects of *"one of the most unanticipated health threats of our time—our increasingly sedentary lifestyles."*

Their argument for movement is the same as mine. *"For thousands of years, that's exactly what humans did. In the mid-20th century, however, rapid technological advances (think: cars, TVs, computers, etc.) began chipping away at physical activity, and as technology did more of the heavy lifting, people became increasingly sedentary."* A 2018 analysis of research by *BMC Medicine* showed a dose-response relationship between the time spent sedentary and all-cause mortality. In short, the more time we spend moving in some way on a regular basis, we decrease our risk of disease and poor health outcomes of any kind.

When we start to move our body regularly, most any health complaint we may have will be likely to improve. And there will be other desirable effects gained, like increased energy and mental clarity.

Stand more during the day and walk around at work. Take breaks and see if your boss will get you a standing desk. At home, come up with alternative activities to sitting down and watching a screen at the end of the day. For exercise, start wherever you're at. Walking is not a bad place to begin, especially if you're not used to regular exercise. My favorite activities to recommend to patients are walking, hiking, biking, high-intensity interval training (HIIT), and power yoga/vinyasa flow. It can also be really helpful to enlist a personal trainer to keep you motivated and prevent injury. When exercising, focus on increasing your heart rate, fatiguing your muscles, and sweating. Aim for 20 to 75 minutes, three to five days a week, depending on the intensity. Muscle-strengthening exercise is important two or more days a week. Check out the CDC for more specifics regarding exercise guidelines and recommendations.

PILLAR 3

Diet

There are so many diets out there; it can be hard to know what to pay attention to, or even where to start. To complicate things further, depending on whom you listen to and what your goals are, there can be wildly differing and opposing opinions. I prefer a simple structure with a few easy to understand elements. These guidelines cover the most essential aspects of a healthy diet.

A FOUR-STEP HEALTHY DIET CHECKLIST

☐ Whole foods

☐ Plant-based diet

☐ Clean foods

☐ Variety

This list is the essence of what is termed an anti-inflammatory diet. When we understand each of these steps and implement them in 95 percent of what we put in our body, we will have a diet that is nutrient-dense, high in fiber, anti-inflammatory, and promotes longevity.

Whole Foods

Whole foods are anything that comes straight from the ground or from an animal. These foods are not yet processed into other products. Vegetables, herbs, beans, nuts, and fruits are all examples of whole foods. Cuts of meat and fresh fish or seafood also count. The closer the food is to its original form and harvest, the better it will be for your health.

The closer the food is to its original form and harvest, the better it will be for your health.

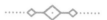

As we move away from a strictly whole foods definition, we still have many healthy options, but it requires more diligence on our part. For example, hummus can be really healthy, depending on what's in it. Hummus should only be chickpeas, olive oil, water, salt, tahini, and lemon juice. Unfortunately, if you start to look at labels, you'll usually find cheap ingredients, like soybean or corn oil and high-fructose corn syrup, as fillers in processed foods. These inexpensive replacement ingredients are a major reason processed foods are detrimental to our health. If we eat whole foods, things get simpler, as there's no ingredient list to consider in the first place.

Plant-Based Diet

Some people really love their meat. If this is you, fear not. You don't have to be a strict vegetarian to eat healthy. However, I suggest the majority of food going into your body be of plant origin (i.e., vegetables, beans, nuts, seeds, etc.). Plants are where we get fiber, a lot of essential vitamins and minerals, and beneficial antioxidants. Ideally, we need to aim for seven to 10 servings of raw, or half servings of cooked vegetables, a day. Start replacing animal products with things like beans and lentils a few times a week. Although there is no exact amount of meat that is best for everyone to consume, people living in "Blue Zones," areas of world with the longest life expectancy, eat about a two-ounce serving (size of a deck of cards) of meat or fish around five times a month. Many people feel very well eating no meat also, such as those on a vegetarian or vegan diet. This Basic Food Guide provides you with a simple starting point to help guide your food decisions.

Clean Foods

"Organic," "pasture-raised," and "wild caught" are a few common terms that can help guide you in decreasing herbicide, pesticide, and other toxin exposures. Eating "clean" is perhaps the most difficult part of the food system to navigate. Foods grown in a conventional agriculture operation are typically laden with chemicals, which are extremely bad for the earth, and us. In humans, many of these chemicals disrupt hormonal, neurologic, and digestive system functions. **They directly cause ill health and chronic illness.** The Environmental Working Group and the Monterey Bay Aquarium Seafood Watch are a couple of helpful resources with information on eating clean and sustainably.

BASIC FOOD GUIDE	
EAT IN ABUNDANCE (MULTIPLE A DAY)	
Vegetables	Lentils
Fruits	Beans
Nuts	Seeds
EAT IN MODERATION/SPARINGLY (5 TO 15 TIMES/MONTH)	
Meat	Dairy
Fish	Whole Grains
AVOID	
Processed Foods	Processed Seed Oils
Refined Carbs/ Grains	Sugar

Abundant information on the regulation, or lack thereof, of various labels, such as grass-fed, humanely raised, etc. is also available with a simple Internet search. You have to do your research, and even then there is often a lot of gray area. We can accomplish clean eating more easily by knowing our farmers. Farmers' markets are an optimal way to support your community as well as personal health. Local food co-ops are another great resource for quality food and information.

Variety

Have you ever heard the phrase "eat the rainbow"? Not only is this smart, but it's also important to eat a mix of plant parts. This means eating roots (beets, parsnips), stems (celery, asparagus), leaves/foliage (kale, cabbage, swiss chard), and seeds (sunflower, pumpkin). It also means not just eating black beans and pinto beans, for example. There are at least a dozen easily accessible types of beans and legumes. Variety is the spice of life, as they say. It happens to also be the vitality of life.

NOTE: *Grains, which I haven't mentioned yet, are hotly debated in the nutrition world. My primary recommendation is if you're eating grains, eat whole grains (whole spelt berries, brown rice, etc.). Eating refined grains, and the kinds of breads we typically find at our grocery stores, are where we find the biggest harmful health effects. Eat whole grains in moderation.*

Nutrition is a massive topic, and there are resources to help you make healthy food decisions in the Resources section (page 188). I strongly recommend visiting some of the websites mentioned there.

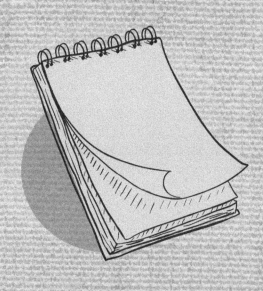

CHAPTER 3

TAKING CHARGE *of* YOUR WELLNESS

One of the most important roles of a good clinician is to be a keen and objective observer. If we're going to help ourselves heal, we need to bring that same level of nonjudgmental objectivity. This chapter is aimed at helping you gain insight into your health, where there may be obstacles to healing, and potential causes of illness. We will lay the framework so that the information in the treatment section can be more successfully applied.

Self-Inquiry and Assessment

Beginning a symptoms log or journal is the best first step toward increasing your awareness. Start by jotting down how you feel in the morning when you wake up, repeating this again at noon, late afternoon, and lastly in the evening. Do this every day. Note your overall energy, how you slept the night before, what your appetite and thirst are like, number of bowel movements, and sense of well-being or lack thereof for each entry.

It's also important to note some specifics about your symptoms. Write these things down as they're happening if possible.

PRIMARY VARIABLES TO NOTE

- Location/sensation of your symptoms (e.g., sharp pain in right temple)
- Time when symptoms arise/go away
- How you were feeling just prior? (Did something tell you it was coming on?)
- Where were you?
- What you were doing?
- How you were feeling emotionally that day or time?

- What makes your symptoms better/worse (moving, cold cloth, eating, etc.)?
- How was your sleep the night before?
- How is your appetite (average, more or less than that)?
- How thirsty are you (average, more or less than that)?
- Do you have any related symptoms (e.g., painful menstrual cramps are the problem, but diarrhea usually happens at the same time)?

Keep this journal for a week. If you only get symptoms once a month, make your journal coincide around that time. Be sure to write down a date and time for each journal entry. This exercise will help you see patterns and give a more accurate picture of your experience than recall typically allows. Doing so also helps you and your practitioners.

This is also a good time to journal honestly in regard to the three pillars we reviewed in chapter 2: mindset, lifestyle, and diet (page 13). On a scale of 0 to 10 (10 being the highest), where do you fall for each one in terms of quality and quantity? What is your level of motivation to change any of those pillars from low/medium to high?

Awareness is the first step to meaningful change. After building awareness, we can begin to look for patterns of potential causation and put our healing treatment plan together.

Set Goals and Intentions

Once you have done some in-depth journaling and reflection, it's time to set your initial goals and intentions. Consider where you would like to start. Think of goals not as an endpoint, but rather a direction you want to move in. Assuming one goal is to be healthy, we're simply trying to consistently make choices that move us in that direction. Set smaller goals for yourself along the way. Perhaps you want to play with your kids or grandkids longer and with decreased pain? Or, you'd like to cook more meals at home? As long as you are moving in that direction, you are meeting your goal consistently. Intention is the mental and emotional energy behind a goal. It's the driving force. Giving spoken and conscious thought to your goals is giving them intention. This is a powerful force when harnessed and focused.

Take your goals seriously but lightly at the same time. Goals require serious intention and attention, but nothing in life is a guarantee. If the goals you set for yourself don't work out as planned, *that is okay*. View it as an opportunity to learn something that will be useful in the future. Contrary to the message our social and cultural constructs give us, success is not the destination—it's in choosing to take the journey.

Creating Your Natural Healing Action Plan

We've covered a lot of ground, and by reaching this point in the book, you have put in the work to more deeply understand your symptoms and overall health. We can now take this information and put it into action. For that, let's establish a **SMARTER** plan of action. This acronym represents long-term goals you can set for yourself as a systematic, step-by-step game plan.

> **NOTE:** *The first five goals, SMART, are done as part of the goal-setting phase. The last two goals, ER, are end-of-the-process checkpoints to review whether you reached your overall health goals. These will help you decide on any changes that need to be made or whether you'd like to create new goals.*

Get SMARTER

Here is an example of a four- to six-week SMARTER action plan, based on a hypothetical initial treatment plan, to get you going on your own goal setting.

SPECIFIC

This is the what, who, why, where, and which of the goal.

EXAMPLE:

What

- *Walk for 30 minutes five days a week*
- *Eat 1 cup of beans four days a week*
- *Take adaptogen tincture and bitters three times a day*
- *Have three more headache-free days over a 30-day time frame*
- *Lose five pounds*

Who Is Involved?
- *My walking buddy*

Where
- *Walking the trails by my house*
- *Eating beans for lunch at work*

Why

- *To be ready for increased cardio next month*
- *To move toward a more plant-based diet*
- *To increase digestion and absorption*
- *To think more clearly at work and with fewer headaches*

Which Resources Are Needed

- *Comfortable walking shoes*
- *Rain coat if the weather is bad*
- *Making lunch the night before work*
- *Timer to remember tincture and bitters*

MEASURABLE

How will you know if you reached your goals? Make sure you can measure your results.

EXAMPLE:

I can easily measure each goal numerically by writing down a tally each night before bed of the daily number met for each goal. I will also be able to tally each day I have a headache.

ACHIEVABLE

Make sure your specific goals are achievable. Are there obstacles in the way of you achieving any of the goals?

EXAMPLE:

I may have a hard time achieving my goal of walking if I have to work late, because that is when I meet my walking buddy. In order to achieve this goal, I will likely need to call them after I get home for encouragement to still go.

RELEVANT

Are your specific goals relevant or in line with your larger, overarching goal?

EXAMPLE:

Yes, all my specific goals relate to my larger goal of losing weight and eliminating headaches.

TIMELY

Put a timeline on your goals. Know when you'll begin, end, and reevaluate. With treatment plans for chronic illness or lifestyle goals, I recommend four- to six-week cycles before reevaluating.

I will start everything in two days, except the beans, which I will start next week, in order to give myself time to buy them and look up recipes. I will meet these goals by week six.

EVALUATE

Objectively decide whether you met your specifications.

EXAMPLE:

- *I walked for 30 minutes four days a week on average instead of five.*
- *I ate 1 cup of beans an average of three times per week instead of four.*
- *I remembered to take my tincture every time, three times a day.*
- *Compared to my last log, I've had three more days of no headaches over the last 30 days.*
- *I lost seven pounds.*

REVIEW AND REFLECT

Decide whether anything needs to change to meet a goal, to set new goals, or if there are any goals to eliminate.

EXAMPLE:

- *I'm okay with my walking amount for now.*
- *I will set a new goal of 1 cup of beans every day, even though I was under my previous goal.*
- *I would like to have the same weight loss and headache reduction in the next six weeks.*

Here is where we cycle back to S. As I already mentioned, for our purposes, I recommend typically giving four to six weeks before reevaluation, as most lifestyle and supportive therapies take time to show effect. At the four- to six-week mark when you reevaluate your goals, also create a new symptom log for at least three days. Comparing the duration, frequency, and intensity of your symptom journal to your previous one is how you'll begin to objectively assess change. Each reevaluation gets compared to the prior symptoms log, and it's helpful over time to compare it to all the previous ones.

Utilize the conditions section to create your initial goals and treatment plan. I recommend starting with no more than three lifestyle changes (one or two is likely more realistic). Behavior change can be difficult, and sustainability is key. In addition to any lifestyle choices you make, I also recommend not exceeding three new things that you choose to take, like herbs or supplements. This recommendation applies to the first treatment plan, but also to each successive modification of the previous plans. Ideally, you're only needing to tweak and refine as you go versus starting new each time. I always recommend working with a trusted health professional when creating your health plans, particularly in regard to supplement decisions.

The Anatomy of Healing

The healing process can look a lot of different ways and take varying amounts of time, depending on the person, the specific condition, and the length of time of the illness. Although rapid improvement and restoration of health does sometimes happen, when dealing with chronic illness, expecting slow and steady improvement with little hiccups along the way is more realistic. It's important not to get too hyper-focused on the day-to-day once you begin a treatment protocol. It's better to look from month to month or every couple of months. Based on your journal entries, if you improved at all over the previous month, that is all that matters. A 10 percent improvement in one month means you'll be feeling amazing in 10 months if you keep that trajectory. If you don't notice any change or feel worse, something in the treatment plan needs to change.

The number one piece of advice I can give when assessing healing from chronic health problems is to *focus on the overall trajectory of things and not the pace.* The only thing that matters is that you're moving in the right direction. Remember to be gentle with yourself and aim for slow but steady improvements.

Moving Toward Freedom

Congratulations on your decision to take health and wellness into your own hands. Reaching out for help, and in this case, reaching for this book, is a vital first step in personal healing as well as helping others. Every moment is a chance to live our lives in a way that's congruent with our values and how we want to exist in the world. Increasing health is experienced as increased freedom in all areas of our lives. Exuberantly go forward and find your freedom. You were born with the magic of healing inside of you. The natural order of the universe is on your side.

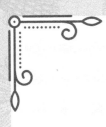

PART TWO

REMEDIES *for* COMMON AILMENTS

With self-inquiry complete and goals set for the diet, lifestyle, and other behavior changes you'd like to implement, we can now dive into natural treatments for common ailments.

With the foundational concepts for natural healing in place, we are in a good place to explore what natural medicine looks like on a deeper level. After we cover the common symptoms, root causes, and testing of each ailment, we'll review effective treatment options to consider. Treatments will focus on specific diet recommendations as well as useful herbal medicine and nutrient supplements. These therapeutic approaches are designed to support the function of important body systems related to the disease as well as addressing likely underlying causes. Affirmations will be given for each condition as a way to increase intention and attention to the healing of the ailment. Lastly, we'll review lifestyle, behavioral, and any other specific treatment approaches to consider.

REMEDIES GUIDANCE

All supplements are given in varying dose ranges and always need to be adjusted appropriately for age, weight, and the individual scenario. The dose ranges given are adult doses and are generally quite safe. Pay attention to overall daily dose in order to not exceed the safe upper limit. For example, if you're taking a multivitamin, it may replace the need for another nutrient recommended, or it may mean a portion of the dose recommendation is covered in the multivitamin.

For some conditions, there are long lists of nutrients. When possible, it's recommended to obtain a quality multivitamin, multimineral, or other supplement product with many of the desired nutrients present in order to avoid having a number of individual pills and to possibly reduce cost as well. At the same time, it often isn't necessary to take every nutrient or herb mentioned to see benefit. The goal in this section is to give the therapeutics for consideration that will likely give the best result. Where herbal formulas are given, try a combination of the herbal formula with the recommended nutrients. Nutrients tend to provide the body with what it needs to function, whereas herbs commonly support those functions to work more optimally. Again, it's recommended to work with a provider who can guide you on the best nutrients and doses for your individual case.

DURATION OF TREATMENT

Some therapies mention how long to take them. For others that don't, a rule of thumb is when you start to see improvements, stick with that regimen for a few months before stopping. The goal is for the body to get what it needs to do the job of healing and ideally not need support any longer. That completely depends on the condition and the individual, however. It may require experimentation to see what works best for you. As mentioned in the disclaimer, please also work with a medical provider for support in this type of decision-making.

MAGNESIUM

When magnesium is listed, either magnesium glycinate or magnesium citrate is the recommendation. Either of these types will be well absorbed.

VITAMIN B COMPLEX

Every B complex has varying doses of each B vitamin and different forms of the vitamins. In general, look for a product that has L-methylfolate instead of just folate, and something that provides the daily dose of each vitamin at the minimum.

MULTIVITAMIN AND MULTIMINERAL

The doses for these all vary. Aim for at least the daily dose of most nutrients and take a serving a day as described on the bottle.

HERBAL FORMULAS

Check with a local herbal shop for the herbal medicines. Many times, they can compound specific liquid formulations for you. If a particular herb isn't available, it can be left out or replaced with an herb of similar action. An herbalist can help you here. The dose ranges given are fairly broad, because some people are more sensitive and need less, whereas others need a higher dose. Experimentation may be necessary to find what works for you.

LAB TESTING AND IMAGING ACRONYMS

Many lab and imaging tests mentioned in the following section are listed as acronyms. Some of the acronyms are listed here for your reference.

ANA – Antinuclear Antibodies

ASCA – Anti-Saccharomyces Cerevisiae Antibodies

CBC – Complete Blood Count with White Blood Cell Differential

CMP – Comprehensive Metabolic Panel

CRP – C-Reactive Protein

CT – Computed Tomography Scan

DHEA-S – Dehydroepiandrosterone Sulfate

ESR – Erythrocyte Sedimentation Rate

fT3 – Free T3 (Triiodothyronine)

fT4 – Free T4 (Thyroxine)

GGT – Gamma-Glutamyl Transferase

hCG – Human Chorionic Gonadotropin

hsCRP – Highly Sensitive C-Reactive Protein

MRI – Magnetic Resonance Imaging

pANCA – Perinuclear antineutrophil cytoplasmic antibodies

RBC – Red Blood Cell

RF – Rheumatoid Factor

SHBG – Sex Hormone Binding Globulin

TSH – Thyroid Stimulating Hormone

tT3 – Total T3 (Triiodothyronine)

tT4 – Total T4 (Thyroxine)

UA – Urinalysis

Please review the Disclaimer on page xii if you're a nonpractitioner.

ADDICTION (SUBSTANCE USE DISORDER)

Symptoms

Common symptoms can be numerous and are largely encompassed in the diagnostic criteria listed in the testing section.

Medically speaking, addiction is categorized into either a substance use disorder (SUD) or a gambling disorder. Here, we're focusing on SUD. With SUD, use and behaviors tend to become increasingly compulsive in nature over time, and the individual will typically continue use despite harmful effects to themselves or others.

Root Causes

Addiction is a complex chronic illness, which is biopsychosocial and spiritual in nature, meaning all of these areas intersect in different and often complex ways to give rise to the holistic picture of what addiction really is as a disease.

Research shows that addiction is a chronic illness of the brain, which involves various circuits, including neurotransmitter and reward system pathways. SUD, as well as other addictions, have interconnections with social and interpersonal relationships, genetic and environmental factors, and mental and emotional characteristics.

Childhood trauma and post-traumatic stress disorder (PTSD) are two areas strongly linked to SUD that should be explored as potential root causes. Ancestral history of SUD and concurrent mental illness are common underlying causes as well.

Addictions can incite feelings of guilt and shame, a loss of sense of purpose and connection to oneself, and a lack of connection to a higher power. Here, a spiritual component often plays a role.

Testing

Two of these 11 conditions need to be present for SUD diagnosis per the *DSM-V*. The more that are present, the more severe the condition.

1. Taking the substance in larger amounts or for longer than you're meant to.

2. Wanting to cut down or stop using the substance but not managing to.
3. Spending a lot of time getting, using, or recovering from the use of the substance.
4. Cravings and urges to use the substance.
5. Not managing to meet goals at work, home, or school because of substance use.
6. Continuing to use, even when it causes problems in relationships.
7. Isolating yourself from social, occupational, or recreational activities because of substance use.
8. Using substances despite the possibility of ending up in dangerous situations.
9. Continuing to use despite having a physical or psychological problem that could be exacerbated by the substance.
10. Increased tolerance, meaning you need more of the substance to get its full effect.
11. Development of withdrawal symptoms, which can be relieved by taking more of the substance.

LABS

- Urine Drug Analysis
- CBC
- CMP

Depending on the nature and length of use, sex hormones (testosterone, estrogen, etc.) and TSH may also be of value.

If someone is using intravenous drugs, regardless of attesting to clean needle use, labs for HIV and hepatitis C should be run.

Treatment

Dietary Approach

A plant-based, nutrient-dense diet is paramount to recovery from SUD. SUD often involves decreased appetite and can easily lead to nutrient deficiencies for this reason and to increased nutrient requirements.

- 50–80oz of water daily
- 7–10 servings of vegetables daily
- 1 cup nuts (almonds, cashews) daily
- Beans and legumes multiple times a week

Herbs/Supplements

For those in post-detox from any substance, it's recommended to take the following:

- Magnesium – 300–600mg daily at bedtime
- Vitamin B Complex – one serving daily
- Electrolyte Powder – one packet/serving in 16oz water daily
- Multivitamin – one serving daily
- Protein powder if undernourished – 1–1.2g/kg of body weight daily
- Fish Oil – 1g one to two times daily

For those in depressant rehabilitation (e.g., recovering from opiate or alcohol abuse) in the first one to three months after detox:

- Glycine – 500–1000mg two to three times daily
- Gamma-Aminobutyric Acid (GABA) – 500mg two to three times daily
- L-theanine – 500mg two to three times daily
- Taurine – 500mg two to three times daily
- Milk Thistle (*Silybum marianum*) – 1,000mg twice daily

The following nutrients are used to calm the nervous system and help with anxiety, restlessness, and sleep. Use them in addition to the nutrients recommended for all substances. Overall mild, safe, and calming herbs include:

- Skullcap (*Scutellaria lateriflora*)
- Passionflower (*Passiflora incarnata*)
- California Poppy (*Eschscholzia californica*)
- Lemon Balm (*Melissa officinalis*)
- Chamomile (*Matricaria recutita*)
- Catnip (*Nepeta cataria*)
- Vervain (*Verbena officinalis*)
- Lavender (*Lavandula angustifolia*)

Stronger herbs for anxiety and insomnia:

- Valeriana (*Valeriana officinalis*)
- Kava Kava (*Piper methysticum*)

ADDICTION RECOVERY HERBAL TINCTURE/GLYCERITE FORMULA

Ashwagandha (*Withania somnifera*)
Bacopa (*Bacopa monnieri*)
Holy Basil, aka Tulsi (*Ocimum sanctum*)
Siberian Ginseng (*Eleutherococcus senticosus*)

Mix equal parts of the four herbs. Take 2–4 droppersful three times daily.

Lifestyle Changes

As difficult as it may be, change your social structure and end friendships with users until they're also clean. Delete all drug supplier contacts from your phone, and work to get into a safe and clean-living environment.

Start exercising as soon as possible after detoxing. You may have to work up slowly in intensity and duration of time, but it will help your brain and body rehabilitate faster. Work with an addiction medicine specialist, seek out counseling and trauma therapy, and attend support groups regularly.

Affirmation

I am a beautiful person, deserving of love and kindness. I live my life with purpose and passion.

ADRENAL EXHAUSTION/FATIGUE

Symptoms

- Feeling "burned out"
- Decreased response to "stressors," e.g., slow reaction time in traffic, slow startle reflex, etc.
- Apathy
- Salt and/or sugar craving
- Depression and/or anxiety
- Frequent illnesses
- Unrefreshing sleep
- Difficulties falling asleep and/or staying asleep
- Generalized fatigue
- Need stimulants to function (Coffee is a common example, and it tends to be less effective over time.)

Adrenal exhaustion, or adrenal fatigue, is not an official medical diagnosis. It's often used to describe a set of symptoms that most closely relate to what one might commonly call "burnout."

The overarching theme, from my clinical experience, is decreased resilience to stressors both internal and external. The individual is so "burned out," they no longer have the vitality to respond to the world in a healthy way.

Root Causes

This condition is functional, as opposed to pathological, which means there isn't a disease present in the common use of the term, but there is decreased function of certain body systems, usually due to overuse and overexertion.

Any prolonged stress over months or years is the most likely root cause. Think of students, caregivers, single parents, etc. Other potential scenarios leading to this might be chronic infections or chronic inflammatory states, which are intense stressors on the body.

Testing

- 24-hour Cortisol Mapping*
- Cortisol Awakening Response
- CMP, Fasting
- CBC
- HbA1C
- TSH
- Ferritin
- DHEA-S

*It is important to use a lab that maps out the cortisol response over a 24-hour period to check whether the pattern is high or low at various points in the day or night. I use dried urine analysis.

Treatment

Dietary Approach

- Increase electrolytes. Use a couple of different types of sea salt when cooking.
- Get at least 1–1.2g/kg body weight of protein daily.
- Get 30–50g of fiber daily.
- Eliminate sugar.
- Decrease caffeine. No more than 1 cup of coffee in the morning. Eliminate caffeine if you're able until recovered.
- Drink 50–80oz of water daily.

Herbs/Supplements

- Magnesium – 300–600mg daily at bedtime
- Vitamin B Complex – one serving daily
- Multimineral – one serving daily

ADRENAL FATIGUE HERBAL TINCTURE FORMULA

Ashwagandha (*Withania somnifera*)
Holy Basil, aka Tulsi (*Ocimum sanctum*)
Schisandra (*Schisandra chinensis*)
Siberian Ginseng (*Eleutherococcus senticosus*)

Mix equal parts of the four herbs. Take 2–4 droppersful three times daily.

Lifestyle Changes

Your body has to get adequate rest in order to repair. In a depleted state, rest and sleep is how your body will have the time to build itself back up. Go to bed by 11 p.m. and get seven to eight hours of sleep a night. If insomnia is a problem, visit that section (page 140) for more guidance.

Start moving your body however you can. Walking vigorously for 15 minutes after dinner is a good place to start. It may feel depleting, so start with what you are capable of and slowly increase, gently pushing your boundaries. Small efforts here will give faster improvement. Remove the obstacles to cure. This means you have to change the situation that is causing or contributing to the exhaustion however possible. Without this, full recovery will be difficult.

Affirmation

I care for myself as lovingly and attentively as I care for others.

Or, I give myself as much love and attention as everything else in my life.

ALLERGIES

Symptoms

- Itchy eyes, ears, nose, and/or palate (roof of mouth)
- Sneezing
- Runny nose
- Watery eyes

- Sinus/nasal congestion
- Headaches (frontal/sinus)
- Postnasal drip
- Occasionally cough or wheeze (if asthma is present)

NOTE: *This description is not related to the topic of food intolerances/sensitivities, which some people call food allergies. This description is in reference to things like seasonal allergies, allergies to other substances like dust mites and animal dander, and "true" food allergies.*

Root Causes

The immune system is reacting intensely to something in the external environment. The IgE (usually pretty reactive) part of the immune system is the most common with acute allergic reactions. This IgE is behind anaphylactic (life-threatening) reactions, but also causes many things like seasonal allergies. When certain immune cells, called mast cells, get triggered in this way, histamine is released. Histamine causes the uncomfortable symptoms we experience.

Testing

Testing is often not necessary for diagnosis. However, if there are problems on a continual basis, versus seasonally, knowing the specific allergen(s) is more important.

- IgE Allergen Panel
- Skin Prick Test
- CBC

Treatment

Helpful treatment approaches include allergen avoidance, optimizing histamine breakdown, stabilizing mast cells (histamine producing cells), and allergy
hygiene.

Dietary Approach

- Eliminate known food intolerances.
- Eat as many bioflavonoid-rich plants as possible.
- Increase intake of foods high in vitamin C.
- Incorporate pumpkin seeds and cashews for increased zinc.
- Eat foods high in quercetin daily.
- Drink 50–80oz water daily.

Local honey is a folk treatment/prevention for pollen allergies. Some studies have
shown benefit and others not. Honey tastes good, is safe for those over one year
old, and may be helpful.

Herbs/Supplements

- Vitamin C – 1000mg one to three times daily
- Vitamin B Complex – one serving daily
- Quercetin – 250–500mg one to three times daily (a general Bioflavonoid
  Complex in place of Quercetin is fine)
- Calendula (Calendula officinalis) and Nettle (Urtica dioica) leaf steeped tea
  a few times daily

Lifestyle Changes

Avoidance of allergens prevents a reaction from happening. Make avoidance the
first priority whenever possible.

With pollen allergies, keeping yourself and your indoor environment as free
from those pollens as possible is key. Taking your clothes off at the door and
having a bag to put them in is one way to avoid tracking in the pollen. At the least,
wash your face and hair before bed. Otherwise, you're taking the pollen to bed
with you.

Dust mites are a common allergen. Get a dust mite cover for your pillow, wash
it often, and replace your pillow every six months for good measure. Keep your
home as dust free as possible. Getting the surfaces damp first will prevent getting

dust in the air when cleaning. Don't forget window blinds; this is a common place for dust to accumulate.

An indoor air filter can be beneficial to keep particulate matter out of the air for any airborne allergens. With airborne allergens of any type, it's important to wash your clothes and sleeping materials often. Pillowcases can be especially important.

Affirmation

I have strong and healthy boundaries with others and my environment.

ALZHEIMER'S DISEASE

Symptoms

Short-term memory loss is the most common first sign of Alzheimer's disease (e.g., misplacing objects frequently, repeating questions, and forgetting what was done earlier in the day like what was eaten for breakfast).

As time and the disease progress, common symptoms are:

- Difficulty with more complex cognitive tasks/problem-solving
- Impaired reasoning and/or judgment
- Confusion of time and place
- Errors in speaking/writing
- Difficulty recognizing objects
- Decreased ability for normal activities of daily living/decreased autonomy
- Behavioral and emotional dysregulation

Root Causes

Alzheimer's Disease (AD) is by far the most common type of neurodegenerative disease. It's a sporadic type that has onset in older age, typically after age 65, and is usually slowly to moderately progressive.

Buildup of beta-amyloid plaques and tau proteins, which cause neurofibrillary tangles, affect nerve transduction and play a role in the degeneration of surrounding neurons. Although these are associated with the degeneration and directly cause some of the symptoms, there are much deeper questions that should be asked as to why this disease occurs in the first place.

Putting aside predispositions due to inherited genes, behavioral and environmental factors are left to consider. Major considerations for AD from a naturopathic perspective are:

- Gut dysbiosis and pathogens
- Leaky gut/intestinal permeability
- Heavy metal toxicity (e.g., aluminum, mercury)
- Other toxin burden (pesticides, herbicides, etc.)
- History of inflammatory behaviors, including:
  - Smoking
  - Heavy alcohol use
  - Pro-inflammatory diet

- Chronic infections (e.g., Borrelia, Epstein-Barr virus)
- Leaky blood-brain barrier (resulting in neuroinflammation)
- Nutrient deficiencies

Testing

There is no established lab or image testing to confirm the presence of AD.
A thorough neurologic and mental status exam should be performed. Doing so
helps rule out other conditions and other types of dementia. Labs can help rule
out other causes of presenting symptoms, such as infections or other organ
pathology.

- CBC
- CMP
- TSH
- Methylmalonic Acid
- CRP
- ESR
- Neutrophil/Lymphocyte Ratio (NLR)
- Lipid Panel
- Vitamin D
- ANA with Reflex Cascade
- Iron Panel with Ferritin
- RBC Magnesium

Other Considerations

- Urine Toxic Metals Screen
- Comprehensive Stool Analysis
- Comprehensive Nutrient Panel
- Genetic SNP Panel
- Testing for Pathogens – Reactivated Epstein-Barr Virus and Cytomegalovirus Virus, Lyme Disease, and other tickborne diseases, particularly if there's a history and other tests aren't showing much.
- Brain MRI to look for other brain disorders

Treatment

Conventional treatment is to give acetylcholinesterase inhibitors. The *Merck Manual* states these medications "modestly improve cognitive function and memory in some patients." Although there may be herbs that potentially help preserve choline through similar actions, we need to move beyond thinking too reductionist. The greatest efficacy in chronic conditions comes from a more holistic approach and treating any underlying contributing factors. Hence, the broad testing recommended here.

Dietary Approach

The primary importance is to stay nourished, especially if decreased appetite and difficulty remembering to eat are present. An anti-inflammatory diet is the basis for improving brain inflammation and getting the nutrients needed for brain function.

- 30–50g of fiber daily
- 50–80oz water daily
- At least 1–1.2 g/kg body weight of protein daily
- 7–10 servings of vegetables daily

Some have proposed a ketogenic diet may be beneficial. There is minimal human research available, especially long-term evidence, and this diet can be difficult to maintain, even for a healthy person. It's not likely the best first place to put your energy, but it may be worth consideration after getting some of the other treatments on board and giving them due diligence.

Herbs/Supplements

- Vitamin B Complex – one serving daily
- Magnesium – 300–600mg daily
- Acetyl-L-Carnitine – 2–3g daily
- High EPA/DHA Fish Oil – 1g two to three times daily
- Broad Spectrum Probiotic – 5–25 billion CFU by mouth daily
- Electrolyte Powder in 16oz water daily
- Curcumin – 2–4g daily
- Bacopa (*Bacopa monnieri)* – 1000mg once daily
- Dandelion *(Taraxacum officinale)* Root Tincture – 2 droppersful three times daily

BRAIN BLOOD FLOW HERBAL TINCTURE FORMULA

Rosemary (*Rosmarinus officinalis*)
Gotu Kola (*Centella asiatica*)
Ginkgo (*Ginkgo biloba*)

Mix equal parts of each herb. Take 2–4 droppersful two to three times daily.

Lifestyle Changes

Optimize sleep without using sleep medications. These medications increase the risk of falls and create decreased function in an already underfunctioning brain.

Movement is quite important. Depending on the level of disease' severity, anything from walking to chair exercises may be all that is possible. Focus on what is doable and safe. Anything is better than nothing.

Exercising the brain is a good way to keep it functioning well for longer. Do things like puzzles, Sudoku, and crosswords. Be creative: Try drawing, coloring, playing music, writing letters, practicing origami, or whatever is manageable. These kinds of activities obviously vary widely based on disease progression. The point is to stay engaged in activity and avoid stagnation. Neurofeedback is showing promise for cognitive decline in dementia; it's easy to do, and is also like exercise for the brain.

Affirmation

I release the past, live in the present, and engage the world to my full potential.

ANEMIA

Symptoms

- Pallor (pale skin, lips, gums, and conjunctiva)
- Shortness of breath
- Fatigue
- Generalized weakness
- Syncope (fainting)
- Chest pain
- Vertigo
- Headache
- Amenorrhea
- Decreased libido
- Heart palpitations

Root Causes

Anemia is a decrease in red blood cells in circulation and the causes are vast. Blood loss is one cause, in which case the source of the bleeding must be identified. Blood loss in stool is a common cause here.

Decreased red blood cell production is a typical reason for anemia. Iron, B_{12}, folate, and copper deficiencies all cause anemia. Chronic inflammatory disorders and certain cancers can also cause anemia.

Another cause of anemia can be that the red blood cells in circulation are being broken down, or lysed. Things like infections, enlarged spleen, and autoimmune conditions can cause anemia.

Anemia is always a sign of deeper causes to be uncovered.

Testing

The exact kind and cause of anemia must be elucidated through testing. CBC shows the presence or lack of anemia, because it shows the number of red blood cells present as well as their size and the amount of hemoglobin present.

Based on what the CBC shows, it narrows down the choices for the next step. There are whole testing algorithms to help physicians diagnose the specific anemia present.

Treatment

It's important to be a detective with anemia. Once the type of anemia is figured out, keep asking why. For example, if there is a nutrient deficiency, we must understand why that took place and treat that if we are to actually heal the deeper issues involved and not just replace the nutrient with no questions asked.

Dietary Approach

In general, a nutrient-dense, whole-food, and plant-based diet, personalized for your condition, can typically address the underlying nutrient causes of anemia.

Herbs/Supplements

When deficient in a nutrient, repletion with at least the RDA and going to the safe upper limit for a short duration will help expedite improvement. If nutrient depletion is severe, intramuscular or intravenous nutrient repletion is the best course of action, followed by oral supplementation until no longer deficient.

Herbs, supplements, and other treatments need to be tailored to support the affected body systems and pathology involved in the underlying cause of the anemia.

For example, if absorption of a nutrient such as B_{12} is a problem, take digestive bitters and digestive enzymes, for one to three months before meals as well as B_{12} supplementation.

Lifestyle Changes

Assess what behaviors and personal choices may have contributed to the underlying reason for the anemia. The self-inquiry in chapter 3 can help guide you.

Affirmation

I build and maintain life force with ease.

ANXIETY & PANIC ATTACKS

Symptoms

- Restlessness
- Irritability
- Worry, fear, and/or panic
- Muscle aches, pains, and tension
- Chest pain
- Palpitation and/or racing heart
- Difficulty concentrating
- Abdominal pain
- Decreased or increased appetite
- Sleep disturbance
- Shaking/trembling
- Shortness of breath
- Sense of choking/difficulty breathing
- Behaviors like wringing hands or nail biting

Anxiety can manifest physically, mentally, and/or emotionally. The symptoms listed here are typical, but nearly any symptom can be related to, or exacerbated by, anxiety.

Anxiety usually gives an underlying feeling of unease or fear and can range from mild to severe panic disorders.

Root Causes

A large number of health conditions can be the cause of anxiety. According to Medscape.com, "Anxiety disorders have one of the longest differential diagnosis lists of all psychiatric disorders." This is definitely my clinical experience as well.

Different hormonal (hyperthyroid) and metabolic imbalances (diabetes) can cause anxiety. Other potential causes are nutrient deficiencies and/or imbalances, infections, and sleep disorders. Substance abuse, dependence, and withdrawal are also causes for consideration.

When other medical problems are ruled out, generalized anxiety disorder (GAD) is the common diagnosis. To truly diagnose an anxiety disorder, other medical causes have to be ruled out.

Other psychological disorders such as personality disorders and schizophrenia can have anxiety as part of their manifestation.

What can confuse the picture of root cause in anxiety is that *symptoms caused by anxiety can also sometimes be the cause of anxiety.* For example, anxiety can cause heart palpitations. Heart palpitations can also cause anxiety and be present for separate reasons. Tricky, right? I once had a patient who was having heart palpitations and had strong anxiety during them. I wasn't sure if she was possibly having palpitations due to anxiety. As it turns out, this patient was iron deficient and anemic. Addressing the anemia resolved her heart palpitations and her anxiety along with it.

> **NOTE:** *Consider dysfunctional breathing as a commonly overlooked cause of GAD. This condition can easily be treated using biofeedback and breath training.*

Testing

Physiologic and biochemical causes such as hyperthyroidism must be ruled out. A 2018 meta-analysis in *The Journal of the American Medical Association* found that 30 percent of anxiety cases also have autoimmune thyroiditis. A thorough history should guide the tests to be run. Here are some basic starting points.

- CBC
- CMP, Fasting
- TSH

Other Considerations

- 24 Cortisol Mapping*
- Urine Drug Screen
- Urinalysis, Dip Stick
- HbA1C
- Comprehensive Nutrient Panel

I strongly recommend taking the Nijmegen Questionnaire if you have GAD (see the Resources section on page 188). This questionnaire is a quick rating of certain symptoms related to dysfunctional breathing that can cause anxiety, and is treatable.

---

*It's important to use a lab that maps out the cortisol response over a 24-hour period, instead of simply giving you the total amount for the 24 hours. This is because you want to see what the pattern is and whether it is high or low at various points in the day or night. I use dried urine analysis.

Treatment

This treatment approach is in regard to GAD. Other diagnoses need to be treated accordingly.

Dietary Approach

Avoid big spikes and drops in blood sugar. This means avoiding refined sugar and carbohydrates. Eat some protein with each meal, and if blood sugar drops are common, keep some almonds or other nuts with you at all times in order to snack regularly.

- Reduce or eliminate caffeine.
- Reduce alcohol consumption.

Herbs/Supplements

- Magnesium – 150mg–300mg twice daily
- Glycine – 500-1000mg two to three times daily
- GABA – 500mg two to three times daily
- L-theanine – 500mg two to three times daily
- B6 – 10mg daily (a Vitamin B Complex may suffice here as well)
- Taurine – 500mg two to three times daily

All of these nutrients act to help calm the nervous system.

The herbal allies for anxiety are many. If you have anxiety, make them your friends.

Mild, effective, and generally very safe herbs include:

- Skullcap (*Scutellaria lateriflora*)
- Passionflower (*Passiflora incarnata*)
- California Poppy (*Eschscholzia californica*)
- Lemon Balm (*Melissa officinalis*)
- Chamomile (*Matricaria recutita*)
- Catnip (*Nepeta cataria*)
- Vervain (*Verbena officinalis*)
- Lavender (*Lavandula angustifolia*)

Stronger herbs*:

- Valerian (*Valeriana officinalis*)
- Kava Kava (*Piper methysticum*)

*Consult with a practitioner with knowledge of herbs before using these herbs if you're taking other sedative medications as these can amplify the effects.

Cannabis spp. are beneficial for some, but they can also exacerbate anxiety. This herbal medicine is not a typical clinical approach I use for anxiety, but if you are going to try it, I recommend avoiding concentrates like "dabbing." Cannabidiol (CBD) does not create a "high," and is the best place to start. CBD and tetrahydrocannabinol (THC) in a ratio of 20:1 is a reasonable starting place for experimenting with increasing THC amounts. CBD will be more likely to be helpful if it's a full-spectrum product versus only CBD.

Lifestyle Changes

Anxiety lives in the past, and in the future. Learning how to bring your focus to the present moment is paramount. Start practicing getting out of your head and into your body. Begin a daily mindfulness meditation commitment. At the least, sit for 10 to 15 minutes every day in a calm and quiet space and just be. Eliminate all distraction, sensory stimulation, and focus on your body and sensation.

Biofeedback and heart rate variability training will help balance the nervous system, prevent anxiety, and help stop anxiety attacks in the moment.

Also, take time to be in nature on a regular basis.

Affirmation

My feet are planted. I am here, now, in this moment. I am safe in my body.

Asthma

Symptoms

- Chest tightness/constriction
- Shortness of breath/rapid breathing
- Racing heart
- Wheezing
- Mucus production in airways
- Cough

Mild asthma will usually be asymptomatic unless triggered. More severe illness will present with more intense symptoms, symptoms between exacerbations, and oftentimes symptoms in the middle of the night.

Root Causes

Immune system imbalance and inflammation underlie asthma. There is a sensitivity of the airways. The inflammatory immune processes underway when triggered cause the airways to become constricted. Common triggers are cold air, exercise, emotional excitement, infection, seasonal/environmental allergies, acid reflux, and aspirin and other NSAIDs.

An important underlying problem to evaluate is food intolerance. It has long been observed that atopic dermatitis (eczema) and asthma are commonly found together. Food intolerances can underpin both of these conditions. Systemic inflammation may also be present with asthma presentations.

Testing

- Pulmonary Function Tests
and/or
- Peak Flow

Either of these tests should be done, if possible, using a bronchodilator like Albuterol to assess before and after administration.

- CBC
- IgE Allergy Panels for foods, pollens, dust, etc.
- CRP
- Neutrophil/Lymphocyte Ratio (NLR)
- Food Elimination/Re-Challenge to assess for intolerances/sensitivities

- IgG Food Allergy Test
- Chest X-ray
- Assess for acid reflux

Treatment

In acute episodes, bronchodilation is imperative. Mucus expectoration is also important.

In the long term, immunomodulation, decreasing inflammation, and improving overall wellness through lifestyle factors are the primary focus.

Dietary Approach

- Follow an anti-inflammatory diet.
- Avoid sugar.
- Eat high bioflavonoid content daily (7–10 servings of vegetables daily, in particular dark purples and brightly colored ones).
- Eliminate food intolerances. This can sometimes render asthma a nonissue.
- Increase intake high vitamin C foods.
- Eat foods high in quercetin daily.

Herbs/Supplements

- Vitamin A – 1500–3000mcg daily
- Vitamin E – 250mg daily
- Vitamin C – 1g two to three times daily
- Selenium – 100mcg daily
- N-Acetylcysteine – 600mg twice daily
- Quercetin – 250–500mg one to three times daily
- Fish Oil – 1g daily
- Curcumin – 1–2g daily

CHRONIC ASTHMA HERBAL TINCTURE FORMULA 1 (AIRWAY SUPPORT & TONIC)

Khella (*Ammi visnaga*)
Elecampane (*Inula helenium*)
Yerba Santa (*Eriodictyon californicum*)

Mullein (*Verbascum thapsus*)
Fennel (*Foeniculum vulgare*)
Ginger (*Zingiber officinalis*)

Mix 25% Khella, 20% Elecampane, 20% Yerba Santa, 20% Mullein, 10% Fennel, 5% Ginger. Take 2–4 droppersful two to three times daily.

CHRONIC ASTHMA HERBAL TINCTURE FORMULA 2
(IMMUNOMODULATING)

Astragalus *(Astragalus membranaceus)*
Siberian Ginseng *(Eleutherococcus senticosus)*
Devil's Club *(Oplopanax horridus)*
Ashwagandha *(Withania somnifera)*
Licorice *(Glycyrrhiza glabra)*

Mix 25% Astragalus, 25% Siberian Ginseng, 20% Devil's Club, 20% Ashwagandha, 10% Licorice. Take 2–4 droppersful two to three times daily.*

> **NOTE:** *Acute asthma attacks are serious and can be life-threatening. Although there are herbal and IV nutrient approaches to treat these acute situations, they are beyond the scope of this book. I always recommend having a bronchodilating medication on hand, even when using natural therapies for asthma. These and other medications can be lifesaving, whereas natural medicine best shines by addressing the underlying causes in order to reduce acute episodes and severity. Never stop asthma medications without guidance from your doctor.*

*These formulas are not designed for treating acute asthma attacks. They are aimed to balance and strengthen the whole system, reduce airway sensitivity, and reduce acute exacerbations and long-term need for medications.

Lifestyle Changes

Follow the recommendations for allergies if present. Doing so will help prevent triggering aggravations of the airway.

Learn nervous system calming techniques like those mentioned in the anxiety section (page 50). Also learn how to diaphragmatically breathe, which is essentially breathing into the belly and the sides of the low ribs instead of the upper chest.

Affirmation

I have strong and healthy boundaries with others and my environment.

ATTENTION-DEFICIT/ HYPERACTIVITY DISORDER (ADHD)

Symptoms

There are three categories of ADHD symptoms:

1. Difficult concentration/inattention
2. Hyperactivity
3. Impulsive behaviors

These symptoms can lead to a variety of problems, such as:

- Trouble staying on task, being present in conversations, playing, etc.
- Trouble staying organized or trouble with time management
- Losing things often
- Easily distracted
- Seeming like the person is not listening
- Difficulty with details
- Restlessness/squirming/fidgeting
- Constant motion and/or talking
- Impatience
- Interrupting

Root Causes

ADHD manifests in childhood but can also carry on into adulthood. It's a neuro-behavioral disorder. Genes, environmental factors, nutrient status, and *in utero* and newborn health such as low birth weight and head injuries are all potential causes and contributing factors for this condition.

Root causes to consider are anything that can affect neurodevelopment or neurobiology of an individual.

Testing

- CBC
- CMP, Fasting

- TSH
- Methylmalonic Acid
- Ferritin
- Neutrophil/Lymphocyte Ratio (NLR)
- RBC Magnesium
- Zinc
- Urine Toxic Metals Screen
- Consider Comprehensive Stool Analysis
- Consider a Comprehensive Nutrient Panel
- Consider Genetic SNP Panel
- Food Elimination/Re-Challenge to assess for intolerances/sensitivities

Treatment

Treat any underlying nutrient deficiencies or other findings appropriately, in addition to these recommendations.

Dietary Approach

- Eliminate sugar and processed foods.
- Focus on nutrient-dense, whole foods.
- Eat organic, at least the Dirty Dozen by the Environmental Working Group (EWG), as well as wheat and oats.
- Eliminate food intolerances.
- Ensure adequate protein, at least 1g/kg of body weight.
- Ensure adequate fiber, at least 30g daily (for those over age 10).
- Ensure adequate hydration.
- Eliminate fruit juices.

Herbs/Supplements

- Fish Oil
- Broad Spectrum Probiotic
- Vitamin B Complex
- Magnesium
- Zinc* (with improvement, taper after three months and reassess without)

No good test exists for reliable zinc evaluation. Even if serum tests come back normal, it may be worth a try to supplement with zinc anyway. With long-term zinc supplementation, you have to also supplement with 1–3mg/day of copper to avoid zinc-induced copper deficiency.

A quality children's multivitamin can cover some of these bases.

All supplements need to be dose-adjusted to age appropriate amounts, which is why doses are left blank, since many of these patients are children.

HYPERACTIVITY HERBAL TINCTURE/GLYCERITE FORMULA

Milky Oats (*Avena sativa*)
Chamomile (*Matricaria recutita*)
Skullcap (*Scutellaria lateriflora*)

Mix 50% Milky Oats, 30% Chamomile, 20% Skullcap. Take 2 droppersful two to three times daily.

Also look at the mild herbs listed in the anxiety section (page 50). These herbs are often helpful for children and can be incorporated into a formula like the one above.

Lifestyle Changes

Decrease screen time to no more than an hour a day. This includes video games, TV, and phones. Avoid shows with rapid shot changes. Stick to entertainment like music concerts, nature, etc.

Get children outside for hikes, playing in the yard, etc. every day if possible. Get them into the woods and water often. Gardening is another grounding outdoor activity for any age. Guide children into creative outlets. Find something they enjoy and feed it.

Biofeedback and neurofeedback are helpful approaches to consider. Consult with a behavioral medicine physician.

Parent Training in Behavior Management (PTBM), as well as training for the teachers involved with the child, will help in managing behavioral difficulties with children. It's ideal to have everyone involved with the child's care aligned on behavioral approaches.

Affirmation

I live at the same speed as the trees, clouds, water, and the bees.

AUTISM SPECTRUM DISORDER

Symptoms

The four primary areas affected are:

- Development
- Social skills/interactions
- Communication abilities
- Learning

The potential symptoms of autism spectrum disorder (ASD) are numerous, and as the name implies, there is a spectrum of severity, types of symptoms, and the impact it has on the person's life.

The symptoms of ASD start before age three. There are sometimes differences noticed in infancy, but even with initially normal development, 80 to 90 percent of parents start to see problems arising by age two.

Behaviorally, individuals with ASD may have repetitive behaviors in speech or action. There can be obsessive interests as well as extreme organization.

Speech and communication problems can be things like giving unrelated answers to questions, children not pointing at objects or responding to pointing as a form of identification, talking monotone or in a sing-song voice, and not understanding joking or sarcasm.

Children with ASD can be exceptionally gifted in terms of intelligence, and there can also be severe disability. This fact is an example of the individuality possible within this condition.

The CDC lists possible red flags as:

- Not responding to their name by 12 months of age
- Not pointing at objects to show interest by 14 months
- Not playing "pretend" games (pretend to "feed" a doll) by 18 months
- Avoiding eye contact/wanting to be alone
- Trouble understanding other people's feelings/talking about their own feelings
- Delayed speech/language skills
- Repeating words/phrases over and over
- Giving unrelated answers to questions
- Getting upset by minor changes
- Obsessive interests
- Flapping their hands, rocking their body, or spinning in circles
- Having unusual reactions to the way things sound, smell, taste, look, or feel

See a resource like the CDC or the National Autism Association online for a more comprehensive symptom list.

Root Causes

ASD is a neurodevelopmental disorder. Genetic and environmental components both appear to play prominent roles. Much like what is written here about ADHD (page 58), anything that effects neurodevelopment such as genetics, environmental factors like heavy metal toxicity, nutrient status, and in utero and newborn health like low birth weight are all possible contributing factors. Interestingly, traumatic brain injuries and autism both share similar characteristics and may hold future keys to learning causes and treatment.

Testing

If there is concern about ASD, a comprehensive evaluation is recommended. Specialists like pediatric neurologists, pediatric psychiatrists, and pediatric developmental specialists are all options.

Besides a specialized evaluation to see if a child meets ASD diagnostic criteria, there should be questioning about environmental toxicity exposures, family history, and the mother's health during pregnancy.

- CBC
- CMP
- TSH
- Neutrophil/Lymphocyte Ratio (NLR)
- Methylmalonic Acid
- Ferritin
- RBC Magnesium
- Zinc
- Urine Toxic Metals Screen
- Food Elimination/Re-Challenge to assess for intolerances/sensitivities
- Comprehensive Stool Analysis (optional)
- Comprehensive Nutrient Panel (optional)
- Genetic SNP Panel (optional)
- Urine Organic Acids (optional)

Treatment

Treat any underlying nutrient deficiencies or other findings appropriately. The testing and treatment considerations are essentially the same between ASD and ADHD due to the neurodevelopmental and neurobehavioral context of both.

Dietary Approach

- Eliminate sugar/processed foods.
- Focus on nutrient-dense, whole foods.
- Eat organic, at least the EWG's Dirty Dozen, plus wheat and oats.
- Eliminate food intolerances.
- Ensure adequate protein, at least 1g/kg of body weight.
- Ensure adequate fiber, at least 30g daily (for those over age 10).
- Ensure adequate hydration.
- Eliminate fruit juices.

Herbs/Supplements

- Fish Oil
- Broad Spectrum Probiotic
- Vitamin B Complex
- Magnesium
- Zinc* (with improvement, taper after three months and reassess without)

All supplements need to be dose-adjusted to age appropriate amounts, which is why doses are left blank, since many of these patients are children.

Lifestyle Changes

Follow the advice pertaining to ADHD on page 58.

Guide children into creative outlets. Coloring, playing music, painting, practicing origami, building with blocks, etc. Find something they enjoy and feed it.

Please note that no good test exists for reliable zinc evaluation. Even if serum tests come back normal, it may be worth a try to supplement with zinc anyway. With long-term zinc supplementation, you have to also supplement with 1-3mg/day of copper to avoid zinc-induced copper deficiency. A quality children's multivitamin can cover some of these bases.

Create a good management team. Seek out a practitioner who specializes in ASD. Obtain teacher and coach reports to help assess any improvements more objectively, beyond the immediate family's observation. Neurofeedback is also a treatment modality worth trying.

Affirmation

Within my uniqueness, I find my light to share with the world.

BENIGN PROSTATIC HYPERPLASIA (BPH)

Symptoms

- Increased urinary frequency and urgency
- Difficulty starting and/or stopping the urine stream
- Increased nighttime urination
- Weak urine stream
- Dribbling of urine
- Pushing in order to urinate
- Incomplete bladder emptying

Root Causes

The word "hyperplasia" in BPH means that there is an increased number of cells. With more cells, the prostate starts to enlarge. The prostate sits right under the bladder and the urethra passes through it, so this enlargement leads to most of the urinary symptoms listed above. There is a physical restriction to outflow of urine that also starts to cause problems in the bladder, leading to worsening urinary retention.

In some respects, BPH appears to be a normal part of aging. By age 85, 90 percent of men have some evidence of cellular changes congruent with BPH. Testosterone possibly plays a role in BPH development also. Testosterone can be converted in the body to a more potent form, called dihydrotestosterone (DHT). It's possible that this DHT is stimulating the changes seen in BPH. However, since testosterone wanes with age, this hypothesis is in question.

Testing

- CBC, to screen for infection
- CMP
- UA, Dipstick
- Urine Culture if infection is suspected
- Prostate Specific Antigen (PSA)
- Ultrasound
- MRI (if necessary, after ultrasound)

Other Considerations

- Sex Hormone Panel
- Bladder Emptying Study

Treatment

Dietary Approach

- Increase bioflavonoids as much as possible.
- Consume quercetin-rich foods daily.
- Increase phytosterol intake.
- Pumpkin seeds are beneficial for the prostate due to phytosterols, zinc, and the seed oil. Pumpkin seed butter is one option to incorporate this into your diet.

Herbs/Supplements

- Stinging Nettle Root (*Urtica dioica*) – 300–500mg daily
- Saw Palmetto (*Serenoa repens*) – 500–1000mg daily
- Beta-sitosterol – 60–100mg twice daily (This supplement is in place of nettle root at this dose, or you can use the two in combination at around half doses each.)
- Zinc* – 15mg daily

URINARY URGENCY AND FREQUENCY HERBAL TINCTURE FORMULA

Skullcap (*Scutellaria lateriflora*)
Wild Yam (*Dioscorea villosa*)
Khella (*Ammi visnaga*)
Black Cohosh (*Actaea racemosa*)

Mix 30% Skullcap, 30% Wild Yam, 20% Khella, 20% Black Cohosh. Take 2-4 droppersful two to three times daily, or at bedtime for nighttime symptoms.

With long-term zinc supplementation, you have to also supplement with 1–3mg/day of copper to avoid zinc-induced copper deficiency.

Lifestyle Changes

Eating a variety of plants and regular moderate to vigorous exercise can make a big difference for BPH symptoms. Sometimes symptoms may be aggravated from activities like riding a bike. If so, choose exercise that does not put pressure on the area.

Affirmation

My energy travels with ease through my feet, into Mother Earth. I am grounded.

CELIAC DISEASE

Symptoms

Classic celiac disease (CD) symptoms include:

- Signs of malabsorption (i.e., failure to thrive in children and weight loss)
- Diarrhea
- Steatorrhea (fat in stool)
- Foul smelling stools

  Nonclassical symptoms are also possible, which include:

- Abdominal pain
- Bloating/distention
- Fatigue
- Headache/migraine
- Peripheral neuropathy
- Infertility
- Nutrient deficiencies (e.g., iron, B_{12}, folate)
- Depression
- Anxiety
- Dermatitis herpetiformis (skin condition)

"There are more than 200 known celiac disease symptoms which may occur in the digestive system or other parts of the body." —Celiac Disease Foundation

CD can also be asymptomatic. Asymptomatic individuals don't have symptoms initially, but experience the long-term effects of untreated CD, including villous atrophy and malabsorption.

Root Causes

There is a 1 in 10 chance of developing CD when present in a first-degree relative. Therefore, there is a strong genetic component present in this disease.

When the susceptibility is present, gluten, which is a protein found in wheat, barley, and rye, sets off an autoimmune reaction. The presence of gluten triggers the immune system to attack the lining of the small intestine. The small intestine has millions of tiny finger-like projections, called villi. These villi enhance absorption due to the great surface area they provide. When the small intestine is damaged in CD, these villi get damaged, which leads to malabsorption. This malabsorption can get extreme when untreated.

Testing

Diagnostic Labs

- Tissue Transglutaminase (tTG)-IgA
- tTG-IgG
- IgA Endomysial Antibody
- Total Serum IgA

Other Related Tests

- Gliadin IgA
- Gliadin IgG
- Human Leukocyte Antigen (HLA) DQ2
- HLA DQ8
- HLA DQA1
- HLA DQB1

The blood labs here should be sufficient to diagnose CD. The other related labs are for individual circumstances, and to know the genetics present.

In order for the blood tests (not genetics) to be accurate, the person *must not* already be on a gluten-free diet.

Testing for secondary effects of untreated/newly diagnosed CD:

- CBC
- CMP
- Fasting Lipids
- Ferritin
- Methylmalonic Acid
- RBC Folate
- RBC Magnesium
- Vitamin D
- Comprehensive Nutrient Panel

NOTE: *Gluten sensitivity unrelated to celiac disease is also possible and is typically tested by elimination and symptom improvement. Also, other autoimmune conditions are associated with CD and should be ruled out if suspected. These include, Hashimoto's thyroiditis, Crohn's disease, and type 1 diabetes.*

Treatment

Dietary Approach

The most important step is the complete and meticulous removal of gluten from the diet. No contamination can happen in order to halt the inflammatory process.

- Eat 7–10 servings of vegetables daily.
- Eat a nutrient-dense, whole-food diet to replace nutrient depletions.
- Avoid refined sugar and processed foods.

  Do these steps for the one to two months after diagnosis:

- Smoothie once daily: 1 pear or apple, 1 cup kale, 3 tbsp hemp seeds, ¼ cup pumpkin seeds, 1 cup blueberries, half to one avocado, nut milk or water, plus any powdered supplements from the list below
- 30–50g of fiber daily (use psyllium husk if you need supplemental support)
- Juice three to four times a week: carrot, lemon, celery, beet, chard/kale/cabbage, ginger

Herbs/Supplements

Be sure to do specific and appropriate nutrient repletion based on deficiencies seen in labs.

- Digestive Enzyme with primary meals
- Vitamin B Complex – one serving daily
- Vitamin D – 2000–5000IU daily
- Magnesium – 150mg three to four times daily
- Trace Mineral Supplement – one serving daily
- N-Acetylcysteine – 600mg two to three times daily
- Vitamin C – 1g two to three times daily
- Calcium – 500mg daily
- Zinc* – 15mg daily
- Selenium – 100mcg
- Iron (if deficient) – 25–50mg daily

Take these for three months and reevaluate with labs.

Ensure all supplements are gluten-free. A quality multivitamin can also cover a number of these nutrients, in order to reduce pill number and potential cost.

With long-term zinc supplementation, you have to also supplement with 1–3mg/day of copper to avoid zinc-induced copper deficiency.

Gut Healing (for one to two months):

- L-Glutamine – 3g two to three times daily
- Broad spectrum probiotic
- Curcumin – 1g twice daily
- Calendula tea – 1 tbsp steeped in 1 cup water one to three times daily
- Digestive bitters 5–15 minutes before meals

Lifestyle Changes

Remove all glutinous products from the home. The family needs to be on board for success here, and it's probably best if everyone makes the change to gluten-free to ensure there is no contamination. Also, start taking your own food and snacks to social gatherings. When eating out, ask what the restaurant's practices are to avoid gluten contamination.

Affirmation

Awareness is key. I am free now that I know what isn't good for me.

CROHN'S DISEASE

Symptoms

- Abdominal pain
- Diarrhea
- Fever
- Anorexia

- Weight loss
- Fatigue
- Nausea

Other signs and symptoms can include:

- Fistula (perianal or intestinal) or fissure
- Intestinal abscess
- Bloody stool and/or rectal bleeding
- Bowel strictures/obstruction
- Anemia

- Malnutrition and nutrient deficiencies
- Joint pain and inflammation
- Uveitis
- Erythema nodosum
- Cholangitis

Crohn's disease also increases the risk of intestinal cancer.

Root Causes

Chronic inflammation of the small intestine characterizes this condition. Crohn's disease is in the category of inflammatory bowel diseases (IBD), which also includes ulcerative colitis. The inflammation tends to be in the small intestine and up to the beginning of the colon, but symptoms anywhere in the gastrointestinal tract, from mouth to anus, are possible.

Autoimmunity and genetics play the largest roles in Crohn's disease. There is also a correlation between celiac disease and Crohn's disease. No other specific causative agents have been found.

Testing

- CBC
- CMP
- GGT
- Fasting Lipid Panel
- Methylmalonic Acid
- Iron Panel with Ferritin

- RBC Magnesium
- Zinc
- Selenium
- Copper
- Ceruloplasmin
- CRP

- ESR
- Vitamin A, D, E, K (Fat-Soluble Vitamins)
- pANCA
- ASCA
- ANA with reflex cascade
- Celiac Disease Panel
- Fecal Lactoferrin
- Fecal Calprotectin

Various comprehensive nutrient panels can cover many of the vitamins and minerals mentioned here. The idea is to broadly screen for nutrient deficiencies.

Other Considerations

- Comprehensive Stool Analysis
- Food Elimination/Re-Challenge to assess for intolerances/sensitivities

Imaging is used depending on the severity and acuteness level and can be diagnostic.

- Colonoscopy or Endoscopy with biopsy
- Abdominal X-ray
- Abdominal CT with contrast
- Abdominal MRI

Treatment

The goal of treatment is remission. The primary therapeutic approaches to reach remission are immunomodulation, anti-inflammatory, nutrient repletion, and stress management.

Dietary Approach

- Support small vessels and gut wall healing by consuming 1–2 servings of dark berries daily.
- Eliminate sugar and processed foods.
- Eliminate food intolerances.
- Ensure adequate protein intake, at least 1–1.2g/kg of body weight.
- Eat smaller meals throughout the day.
- Keep well-tolerated foods stocked and prepared at all times.

Herbs/Supplements

Aside from these recommendations, be sure to do specific and appropriate nutrient repletion based on deficiencies discovered in labs if not covered here.

- Digestive Enzyme with primary meals
- Vitamin B Complex – one serving daily
- Vitamin D – 2000–5000IU daily
- Magnesium – 300mg one to two times daily
- Selenium – 100mcg daily
- Trace Mineral Supplement – one serving daily
- N-Acetylcysteine – 600mg two to three times daily
- Vitamin C – 1g two to three times daily
- Zinc – 15mg daily for two to three months
- Iron (If deficient) – 25–50mg elemental iron daily

Inflammation and Gut Support:

- Curcumin – 2g twice daily for acute flares. 1g one to two times daily for maintenance.
- High EPA/DHA Fish Oil – 1–2g daily
- Butyrate – 200–400mg two to three times daily
- Broad spectrum probiotic
- *Aloe barbadensis* leaf pulp/juice – ¼ cup twice daily to heal lesions from flares
- *Calendula officinalis* tea – 1 tbsp per cup hot water one to three times daily for acute flares
- Digestive bitters – 5–15 drops on the back of the tongue, 5–15 minutes before meals until in remission

ACUTE CROHN'S FLARE HERBAL TINCTURE FORMULA

> Licorice (*Glycyrrhiza glabra*)
> Wild Yam (*Dioscorea villosa*)
> Fennel (*Foeniculum vulgare*)

Mix 50% Licorice, 30% Wild Yam, 20% Fennel. Take 3–5 droppersful three to four times daily. Discontinue after symptoms ease and monitor blood pressure, as licorice at this dose may cause it to elevate. If this happens blood pressure will return to normal after discontinuation. If this creates problems sleeping, decrease the dose or don't take it later in the day.

Astragalus *(Astragalus membranaceus)*
Siberian Ginseng *(Eleutherococcus senticosus)*
Devil's Club *(Oplopanax horridus)*
Ashwagandha *(Withania somnifera)*
Licorice *(Glycyrrhiza glabra)*

Mix 25% Astragalus, 25% Siberian Ginseng, 20% Devil's Club, 20% Ashwagandha, and 10% Licorice. Take 2–4 droppersful two to three times daily.

Lifestyle Changes

Smoking tobacco is highly associated with Crohn's disease. Stopping tobacco use should be on the priority list due to this association and the negative effects on healing and the immune system. Manage stress appropriately. Meditation, heart rate variability training, counseling, yoga, and regularly getting into nature are all ways to shift how stress affects us.

Affirmation

I love and accept myself as I am.

DEPRESSION

Symptoms

The Anxiety and Depression Association of America lists the following common symptoms of depression:

- Persistent sad, anxious, or "empty" mood
- Feelings of hopelessness and pessimism
- Feelings of guilt, worthlessness, and helplessness
- Loss of interest/pleasure in hobbies and activities, including sex
- Decreased energy, fatigue, and feeling "slowed down"
- Difficulty concentrating, remembering, and making decisions
- Insomnia, early-morning awakening, and oversleeping
- Low appetite and weight loss or overeating and weight gain
- Thoughts of death/suicide and suicide attempts
- Restlessness
- Irritability
- Persistent physical symptoms that do not respond to treatment, such as headaches, digestive disorders, and pain for which no other cause can be diagnosed

As you can see from the list above, there are many ways of experiencing depression. They can range all the way from tearful sadness, to lack of hygiene, not feeding oneself, and even suicide.

Root Causes

Depressive disorders are a group of psychological diagnoses, but depression is also a symptom of many other conditions. Heredity is thought to play close to half of the role in the cause of depression, except for depression with onset after the age of 60 (late-onset).

There are various theories about other causation, such as neurotransmitter deficiencies or dysregulation, like serotonin, glutamate, and dopamine. Another theory for the cause of depression is dysregulation in neuroendocrine pathways, like the hypothalamic-pituitary-adrenal (HPA) axis.

Depression can also be in response to a traumatic event, like the loss of a loved one. Importantly, though, grief is not depression. Grieving is healthy. Depression is an unhealthy cycle in which one is stuck in, or easily enters, sometimes for no apparent reason. Many people are simply predisposed to entering depression when life events get increasingly stressful, if they lack community engagement, and so on.

Other important considerations for causes of depression are nutrient deficiencies in vitamins and minerals or amino acids, hypothyroidism, adrenal fatigue, chronic infections like Epstein-Barr virus, sleep disorders, gut dysbiosis, and heavy metal toxicity. Chronic illness in itself can cause depression due to decreased quality of life and the suffering that can accompany it.

Testing

Mental health professionals are typically the most qualified to diagnose the exact depressive disorder based on the *DSM-V*. However, there are additional labs to consider to test for other causes.

- CBC
- CMP
- Lipid Panel
- Methylmalonic Acid
- RBC Folate
- RBC Magnesium
- Ferritin
- Zinc
- CRP
- TSH

Other Considerations

- Urine Toxic Metals
- 24-hour Cortisol Mapping
- Comprehensive Stool Analysis
- Comprehensive Nutrient Panel
- Individual Thyroid Hormones

Treatment

In the absence of obvious causes found in labs, testing these recommendations to see what helps is a good next step.

Dietary Approach

- Eliminate food intolerances.
- Get adequate protein, at least 1–1.2g/kg body weight daily.
- Avoid excessive alcohol intake.

Herbs/Supplements

- Multimineral Supplement – one serving daily
- Vitamin B Complex – one serving daily
- Vitamin C – 1g two to three times daily
- L-Tyrosine – 500–1000mg in the morning
- 5-HTP – 150–300mg two to three times daily

DEPRESSION HERBAL TINCTURE FORMULA

St. John's Wort (*Hypericum perforatum*) *
Siberian Ginseng (*Eleutherococcus senticosus*)
Schisandra (*Schisandra chinensis*)
Passionflower (*Passiflora incarnata*)

40% St. John's Wort, 25% Siberian Ginseng, 25% Schisandra, 10% Passionflower. Take 2–4 droppersful three to four times daily for three months before judging efficacy.

Lifestyle Changes

Getting into nature regularly helps bring internal harmony. Make it outdoors, preferably in a park, the woods, or by water, at least three times a week. Regular exercise is a naturally harmonizing activity as well.

Start a practice of meditation and reflection. Depression is often helped by a shift in perspective and orientation to the world. Commit to at least 10 minutes a day.

Address substance use disorders or other addictions by working with a counselor or other mental health professional.

*St. John's Wort interacts with certain medications like SSRIs. Check for interactions if taking other medications and speak with a knowledgeable provider.

Community and social engagement are essential. Find activities that bring you excitement and joy, and ones that feed your spirit. Then seek out others doing those same activities.

Affirmation

I see the dark and the light in the world and myself. I experience them both with grace and gratitude.

DIABETES, TYPE 2

Symptoms

- Increased thirst
- Increased urination
- Increased appetite
- Peripheral neuropathy
- Fatigue
- Blurry vision
- Erectile dysfunction
- Dark patches of skin

Symptoms depend on the level of hyperglycemia (elevated blood sugar) present and for how long. The symptoms listed here are earlier manifestations of the disease. However, as type 2 diabetes mellitus (DM2) progresses, many other symptoms can present that are related to organ damage subsequent to long-term hyperglycemia, such as serious cardiovascular and kidney disease.

Root Causes

Cells use glucose for energy. Insulin is a hormone that helps regulate glucose levels in the blood and it lets glucose enter cells to be used.

Type 1 diabetes (DM1), which typically shows up in childhood, is an autoimmune condition where insulin-producing cells in the pancreas are destroyed and in turn there isn't enough insulin present in the body.

DM2 essentially has the same problems that arise in DM1, but for a different reason. Glucose can't get into the cells very easily to be used, but it's not that there isn't enough insulin around, at least not initially. The problem is, the cells are desensitized to insulin. The cells are resisting insulin (also known as insulin resistance), so that the end effect is high blood glucose because it can't get inside.

Much of the underlying causes for DM2 are lifestyle related and human creations. The primary causes are obesity, sedentary lifestyle, foods and drinks high in refined sugar (especially high-fructose corn syrup), and environmental toxins of many types, termed diabetogens and obesogens. Hemochromatosis, an iron storage disorder, can also cause diabetes.

Testing

- CMP, Fasting
- Hemoglobin A1C
- Lipid Panel, Fasting
- CBC
- hsCRP
- Urinalysis, Dipstick
- Ferritin
- TSH
- Urine microalbumin

Other Considerations

- Insulin
- C-Peptide
- Urine Toxic Metals Screen

Treatment

Treatment needs to be holistic and focused around addressing all the aforementioned causes. Typically, no one factor leads to DM2. The goal should not solely be appropriate management of blood sugar, but treating the variety of causative factors so that a healthy metabolism results.

Dietary Approach

- Eat a plant-based, clean, whole-food diet, as discussed in chapter 2. Doing so is absolutely necessary to overcoming DM2 without medications.
- Eliminate refined sugar.
- Eat *at least* 1 cup beans or lentils daily, ideally at breakfast.
- Eat small meals more frequently.
- Consume 30–50g fiber daily.
- Eat low glycemic-index and glycemic-load foods to aid in blood sugar control.
- Eat protein and fiber with each meal.
- Avoid processed and fast foods.
- Decrease alcohol consumption.

- Experiment with fenugreek in cooking or even as a supplement. It decreases blood sugar after a meal.
- Avoid BPA. Discard all plastic water bottles and food storage.
- Begin intermittent fasting five to seven days a week (start with a 12:12 protocol, then ease into 16:8).

Herbs/Supplements

- Psyllium husk fiber to supplement if unable to meet the full dietary fiber recommendations.
- Chromium – 200–1000mcg daily
- Multivitamin – one serving daily
- Multimineral – one serving daily
- Vitamin D – 2000–5000IU daily
- Cinnamon – 1g two to three times daily
- Berberine - 500mg one to three times daily

DIABETES HERBAL TINCTURE FORMULA

Siberian Ginseng (*Eleutherococcus senticosus*)
Devil's Club (*Oplopanax horridus*)
Schisandra (*Schisandra chinensis*)
Milk Thistle (*Silybum marianum*)
Gymnema (*Gymnema sylvestre*)
Dandelion Root (*Taraxacum officinale*)

25% Siberian Ginseng, 20% Devil's Club, 15% Schisandra, 15% Milk Thistle, 15% Gymnema, 10% Dandelion Root. 2–4 droppersful three times daily, long term.

Lifestyle Changes

Exercise is your friend with diabetes. Make the commitment to start exercising using your big muscles, like thighs and gluts, and getting your heart rate up. Consider getting a personal trainer to help with accountability and safe form when starting exercise regimens. Losing weight will also give noticeable reductions in blood sugar readings, even with a modest weight loss.

Begin sweating at least three times a week for about 20 minutes in a sauna. Doing this long term, along with the other treatments recommended, will decrease total body burden of toxins, help diabetes, and improve overall health. Without sauna access, a hot bath is another way to get a prolonged sweat.

Consult with a diabetes-specific nutritionist.

Affirmation

Today, I put my health first. My choices help me feel vital and alive.

ECZEMA (ATOPIC DERMATITIS)

Symptoms

Atopic dermatitis (AD) is a skin rash that is typically characterized by:

- Itchy patches on the flexor surfaces (i.e., inside elbows, behind knees) and face or neck, although it can be present anywhere.
- Dry and scaly, or moist and clearly inflamed.

The rash will often start at a very young age, even infancy, and can relapse and remit, sometimes over the course of a lifetime. The skin areas where the AD presents can also be thickened from the continual relapsing.

Secondary bacterial infections are not uncommon, especially in children who scratch excessively.

Root Causes

AD is an immune-mediated condition of the skin. Although there is no scientific consensus of the exact cause, there are two primary theories. One theory is that there is an allergic and overreactive immune system. The other theory is that there is a dysfunction in the skin barrier function. There tends to be an allergic component to AD. It's not uncommon for other allergic disorders like asthma to be present or to show up later in life.

It has long been observed by the natural medicine community that eczema resolves when you treat and heal the gut. This observation points to mechanisms of the immune system and gut inflammation, and possibly leaky gut, playing a primary role. Supporting the liver and organs of elimination/detoxification improve eczema as well. This makes a good argument for overall toxic burden and poor gut health as primary drivers of AD.

Research and clinical practice both also show that food allergy, or intolerance, are sometimes the primary causative factor.

Testing

- CBC
- CMP
- Neutrophil/Lymphocyte Ratio (NLR)
- CRP

- IgE Allergen Panel
- Food Elimination/Re-Challenge to assess for intolerances/sensitivities

Other Considerations

- IgG Food Allergy Test*
- Comprehensive Stool Analysis

Treatment

Dietary Approach

- Eliminate known food intolerances.
- Eliminate refined sugar.
- In breastfeeding children, what the mother is eating can cause AD in the infant. The mother needs to avoid problematic foods and experiment with what foods may be affecting the child.
- Eat fermented foods regularly.

Herbs/Supplements

- Vitamin D – 400–2000IU daily depending on age
- Broad Spectrum Probiotic – daily
- Fish Oil – 1g daily
- Oats – Soothe itchy skin by placing oats in a sock, tying it, and using it in a bath or wet and directly apply on the skin.
- Calendula Cream or Salve – to soothe/heal lesions

ADULT ECZEMA HERBAL TINCTURE FORMULA

Dandelion Root *(Taraxacum officinale)*
Astragalus *(Astragalus membranaceus)*
Schisandra *(Schisandra chinensis)*
Burdock *(Arctium lappa)*

*I don't find these tests to be particularly useful, and therefore rarely order them, but they can sometimes be a helpful road map for foods to eliminate and assess for improvement.

Milk Thistle *(Silybum marianum)*
Licorice *(Glycyrrhiza glabra)*

30% Dandelion Root, 20% Astragalus, 20% Schisandra, 10% Burdock, 10% Milk Thistle, 10% Licorice. 2–4 droppersful two to three times daily.

TOPICAL CALENDULA AND YARROW TEA INFUSION

Make a strong tea, at least 1 tbsp of each herb to a cup of water. This can be placed on the skin with a moistened towel or poured directly into bathwater for soothing and healing. I would use half to one gallon if adding it to bathwater. Extra tea can be stored in the fridge for a couple of days.

Lifestyle Changes

Get sun exposure whenever possible. This usually improves AD, possibly because of increased vitamin D. Climate extremes also can be aggravating and cause flares. Sweating can be aggravating initially to AD, but with regular sweating in a sauna, the condition may start to improve through improved bodily detoxification.

Affirmation

I choose what's good for me on the inside, and I see the results on the outside.

ENDOMETRIOSIS

Symptoms

- Nonspecific tenderness in the pelvis (most common symptom)

Whereas around one-third of women with endometriosis will remain asymptomatic, the rest will experience pain in affected areas.

The ovaries are the most common site. Other commonly affected areas are pelvic, inguinal, lower back, and abdominal. Women can experience digestive symptoms such as bloating, nausea and vomiting, painful bowel movements, and alternating constipation and diarrhea. Other common symptoms are painful intercourse, painful menstrual periods, and heavy and/or irregular menstrual bleeding.

Although more unusual, any tissue can be involved, such as lungs, spine, or kidney.

Fertility problems are common in endometriosis, and the symptoms are often cyclical, coinciding with the monthly hormonal cycle.

Root Causes

The endometrium is the lining of the uterus. In endometriosis, normal and healthy endometrial cells exist outside of the uterus. These external sites of endometrial tissue are where the symptoms arise. The way in which the endometrial tissue gets outside the uterus isn't known. We don't know if they migrate there or if other cells are transforming into endometrial cells.

Either way, the end result is tissue that responds to hormonal cycles and causes microbleeds at the site of the tissue, which leads to inflammation and fibrosis of the surrounding tissue and subsequent pain.

Testing

- CBC to screen for infection
- CMP if liver or kidney function are in question
- Neutrophil/Lymphocyte Ratio (NLR)
- CRP
- Urinalysis, Dipstick to rule out urinary tract infection
- Ultrasound (US)

- MRI if necessary, depending on the ultrasound
- Hormone Cycle Mapping can show irregularities that can be treated

Treatment

Dietary Approach

An anti-inflammatory diet high in antioxidants and bioflavonoids needs to be a priority. Avoid sugar and processed foods at the least, as these are pro-inflammatory.

Herbs/Supplements

- Fish Oil – 1–2g daily
- Vitamin C – 1g two to three times daily
- Vitamin E – 250mg daily
- Curcumin – 1–2g daily
- N-Acetylcysteine – 600mg two to three times daily

ENDOMETRIOSIS HERBAL TINCTURE FORMULA

Chaste Tree (*Vitex agnus-castus*)
Dong Quai (*Angelica sinensis*)
Dandelion Root (*Taraxacum officinale*)
Burdock (*Arctium lappa*)
Black Cohosh (*Actaea racemosa*)
Calendula (*Calendula officinalis*)
Red Root (*Ceanothus americanus*)

30% Chaste Tree, 30% Dong Quai, 10% Dandelion Root, 10% Burdock, 10% Black Cohosh, 5% Calendula, 5% Red Root. 2–4 droppersful three times daily.

Lifestyle Changes

Castor oil packs can help pain due to inflammation and tissue stagnation. Apply these packs over the painful area every day for a week and then periodically each week.

Contrast hydrotherapy can improve circulation and lymph flow in the pelvis. Use the hydrotherapy method, focusing on the pelvic region. Feel free to use the same method for pain in a separate area of the body.

Affirmation

I live in a state of hope and optimism.

EPSTEIN-BARR & OTHER VIRAL INFECTIONS

Symptoms

Epstein-Barr virus (EBV) causes mononucleosis (a.k.a. mono). Typical symptoms of mono include:

- Fatigue, sometimes extreme
- Tonsillitis/sore throat
- Liver enlargement
- Spleen enlargement
- Fever
- Rash

Some people are asymptomatic with EBV infection. Severe complications are possible. These include meningitis, encephalitis, and Guillain-Barré syndrome.

EBV stays in the body after it's contracted and eventually goes dormant, also called latency. In some individuals, especially those with a weakened immune system, EBV can reactivate. The primary symptom is often chronic fatigue. However, all of the symptoms above are possible, as well as other body system problems like heart valve abnormalities and coronary artery aneurisms. EBV is also associated with various lymphomas and lymphoproliferative disorders.

Other Viruses

There are viruses that can affect any part of the body. Symptoms correlate with the organs and body systems involved. For some viruses, our immune system will eliminate them and there'll be no further problems. Others like herpes simplex and varicella zoster can reactivate throughout life and cause illness.

Root Causes

Viruses are transmitted in a variety of ways. EBV is usually transmitted through fluids like saliva, blood, semen, and organ transplant.

Viruses aren't alive in biological terms. They're basically just a container holding some genetic material with no way to replicate or make energy, unlike living cells like bacteria. Viruses replicate by using the host person's cellular machinery to copy its DNA and then assemble itself. Most antiviral medications are aimed at affecting different parts of this replication process.

Testing

EBV Testing

- CBC
- CMP
- EBV Viral Capsid Antigen (VCA) IgM Antibody – Acute Infection
- EBV VCA IgG Antibody – Past Infection
- EBV Nuclear Antigen IgG Antibody – Past Infection
- EBV Early Antigen Diffuse (EA-D) Antibody – Recent or Reactivated
- EBV Quantitative Polymerase Chain Reaction (PCR) – Viral Load

Other Viruses

Some viruses have antibody tests. IgM tests look at current, acute infections. IgG looks at past infections. Others have PCR tests to look at the presence and total amount of virus currently present. Some tests, like for influenza, can be run rapidly in the doctor's office.

Treatment

The focus is building up healthy immunity, and using therapies with immune stimulating and antiviral actions.

Dietary Approach

A good dietary approach when living with EBV or other chronic viral infections is to treat food as medicine, meaning incorporating foods that have anti-inflammatory, antioxidant, and antiviral properties. Following an anti-inflammatory diet accomplishes much of this, which includes:

- Onions and garlic daily
- Dark berries regularly
- Copious bright fruits and vegetables and dark leafy greens

ANTIVIRAL SOUP RECIPE

Simmer onion, garlic, and red pepper flakes for 15 minutes on the stovetop using a whole onion and a whole garlic bulb covered with a couple of inches of water. Add red pepper flakes to tolerance. You can keep the leftovers in the fridge and warm it up each day. This will help acute viral infections and reactivated infections.

Herbs/Supplements

- Vitamin A – 1500–3000mcg daily
- Vitamin C – 1g two to three times daily
- Vitamin E – 250mg daily
- Selenium – 100mcg daily
- Zinc – 15mg daily
- *Andrographis paniculata* capsules – 400mg twice daily (chronic EBV)
- Broad Spectrum Probiotic daily (chronic EBV)

Take these for one to two weeks acutely, and for a minimum of two months with chronic EBV or reactivation. Either stop zinc after two months or supplement with copper at 1–3mg daily if continuing.

ACUTE EBV HERBAL TINCTURE FORMULA

Astragalus (*Astragalus membranaceus*)
Lomatium (*Lomatium dissectum*)•
Olive Leaf (*Olea europaea*)
Licorice (*Glycyrrhiza glabra*)
Milk Thistle (*Silybum marianum*)
Red Root (*Ceanothus americanus*)

25% Astragalus, 20% Lomatium, 15% Olive Leaf, 15% Licorice, 15% Milk Thistle, 10% Red Root. Take 3–5 droppersful four to five times daily.

IMMUNOMODULATING HERBAL TINCTURE FORMULA

Astragalus (*Astragalus membranaceus*)
Siberian Ginseng (*Eleutherococcus senticosus*)
Devil's Club (*Oplopanax horridus*)
Ashwagandha (*Withania somnifera*)
Licorice (*Glycyrrhiza glabra*)

Lomatium has been known to cause an itchy rash that can present over the whole body. Although I haven't seen this in practice with much use, it is a real phenomenon to be aware of. The rash ceases after stopping lomatium.

25% Astragalus, 25% Siberian Ginseng, 20% Devil's Club, 20% Ashwagandha, 10% Licorice. Take 2–4 droppersful two to three times daily.

Lifestyle Changes

With acute EBV, avoid spreading infection by limiting exposure to others, especially activities like kissing and sharing food and drink.

Optimizing sleep is necessary for healthy immune function. Prioritize sleep and be sure to do all you can to optimize the quantity and quality.

It can be difficult, especially if a chronic fatigue picture is present, to move regularly. Although the motivation is difficult and the energy is lacking, doing whatever exercise possible is important for improvement from reactivation.

Avoid suppressing a fever; rarely is it a problem with acute infection. If there is discomfort from a fever, use a cool compress on the neck and head, replacing it once it warms.

Affirmation

I have the resilience to live in balance with the viruses that exist with me.

ERECTILE DYSFUNCTION (ED)

Symptoms

The inability to either attain or maintain an erection that is satisfactory enough to perform sexual intercourse.

Root Causes

The primary causes for consideration with ED are hormonal, vascular, neurological, and psychological.

Low testosterone is the primary hormonal contributor for consideration. The vascular cause is typically atherosclerosis of arteries to the penis, usually secondary to smoking or diabetes. Neurologic disorders that cause ED are stroke, multiple sclerosis, various neuropathies, and spinal cord injuries. Psychological causation includes anxiety, fear of intimacy or sexual performance, and guilt. Finally, many drugs can alter erection capability as well.

If a man can get an erection on his own or spontaneously but has a difficult time with his partner, this is a sign of a psychological causation, since it shows the anatomy works. If there is ED in all of the above, it's likely due to biological causes or a combination of factors.

Testing

- Blood Pressure – Test on three separate occasions to screen for hypertension.
- CBC
- CMP, Fasting
- Lipid Panel
- hsCRP
- Hemoglobin A1C
- Sex Hormone Panel

Other Considerations

- Patient Health Questionnaire (PHQ-9) or Hamilton Depression Rating Scale (HAM-D) to screen for depression
- Generalized Anxiety Disorder-7 (GAD-7) to screen for anxiety
- Color Doppler Ultrasound of penile arteries

Treatment

Once the cause is elucidated, we need to tailor our treatment to that. Some primary approaches are listed here. However, looking to the section for the specific condition will provide deeper therapeutic approaches.

Dietary Approach

For vascular complications such as atherosclerosis, a major shift in diet is typically necessary. Aside from a clean, whole-food, plant-based diet, the main focus should be on foods that support healthy lipid balance and small vessel integrity. Look in the heart disease section (page 116) for further cardiovascular disease diet information.

- Fresh garlic – 2–3 cloves daily for at least three months for lipid balance
- Dark berries – 1–2 servings daily for increased small vessel integrity
- Nuts (e.g., almonds, cashews) – 1–2 servings daily for fiber and lipid balance
- 30–50g fiber daily

Herbs/Supplements

For Vascular Causes:

- Fish Oil – 1–2 daily
- Vitamin C – 1000mg two to three times daily
- Hawthorne Berry (Liquid or Solid Extract) – 500mg two to three times daily

Other treatment options for atherosclerosis are in the heart disease section. Also see the specific conditions for treatment related to anxiety (page 50), depression (page 76), and neurologic causes of ED.

Lifestyle Changes

Quitting tobacco and reducing alcohol consumption are two specific lifestyle factors to change. They're inflammatory, and smoking directly contributes to atherosclerosis. Regular exercise will also benefit ED regardless of the cause. Weight-bearing exercise in particular and building lean muscle mass will help with testosterone production.

Affirmation

I am a warrior filled with vitality and exuberance.

FATTY LIVER

Symptoms

- Fatigue
- Pressure or discomfort in the right upper abdomen

Fatty liver, also known as nonalcoholic fatty liver disease (NAFLD), doesn't typically have symptoms present, except for maybe the two listed above. There are fatty infiltrates present in the liver.

Root Causes

NAFLD is mostly a condition associated with poor diet and lifestyle habits. Incidences are increasing in the United States, presumably due to increases in diabetes, metabolic syndrome, and obesity, which are diseases that lead to NAFLD. Hypertriglyceridemia (elevated blood triglycerides) is also associated with NAFLD. When there are too many of these fats in the bloodstream and/or there is blood sugar dysregulation, it appears as though the body starts to deposit some of those fats in the liver.

Some medications can cause fatty liver, and just as overnutrition can lead to fatty liver, the opposite is also true. Severe malnutrition and starvation diets can also lead to NAFLD.

This increased fat in the liver causes inflammation and oxidative damage to the liver cells. The cells die and the liver will enlarge, just as it does with alcoholic fatty liver. Over time, the liver can become fibrotic and undergo cirrhosis from NAFLD.

Testing

- CBC
- CMP, Fasting
- Fasting Lipid Panel
- hsCRP

- Hemoglobin A1C
- Hepatitic C Antibody
- Iron Panel with Ferritin

Liver ultrasound can see fatty liver and a biopsy can tell the difference between fatty liver caused by alcohol or not.

Treatment

Dietary Approach

Visit and follow the diabetes section (page 80) for more information regarding dietary approaches, as these will directly apply to NAFLD. Aside from those recommendations, here are a few more specifics:

- Eat Brassica family plants regularly.
- Eat beets regularly.
- Eat onions and garlic daily if possible.
- Eliminate fructose and other refined sugar.

The liver is the primary detoxifying organ of the body. It has a hard time doing its job when burdened with NAFLD. Eat organic wherever possible to reduce toxin exposure.

Although it's a high-fat diet, a ketogenic diet may decrease NAFLD if the daily calories do not exceed the energy expenditure.

Herbs/Supplements

- Vitamin B Complex – one serving daily
- Magnesium – 300–600mg daily
- Taurine – 500mg two to three times daily
- N-Acetylcysteine – 600mg two to three times daily
- Milk Thistle – 1g two to three times daily
- L-Carnitine – 500–1000mg twice daily

Visit the diabetes section (page 80) for additional supplement and herb information that will be useful in improving blood sugar regulation.

NAFLD HERBAL TINCTURE FORMULA

Dandelion Root (*Taraxacum officinale*)
Artichoke Leaf (*Cynara scolymus*)
Turmeric (*Curcuma longa*)
Licorice (*Glycyrrhiza glabra*)
Red Root (*Ceanothus americanus*)

Mix 30% Dandelion Root, 30% Artichoke Leaf, 25% Turmeric, 10% Licorice, 5% Red Root. Take 2–4 droppersful three times daily.

Lifestyle Changes

Much like diabetes, NAFLD requires an overhaul of diet and lifestyle factors. Weight loss is necessary; although, I find making that the focus is less effective than focusing on healthy eating and exercise. Again, read the diabetes section and that will help you here. Exercise at least a few days a week and incorporate some kind of movement daily.

Affirmation

I have the power to change my health and how I feel. I make decisions that move me in the direction I want to go.

FIBROCYSTIC BREASTS

Symptoms

- Swollen or full feeling breasts
- Painful lumps of breast tissue

The tissue changes with fibrocystic breasts (FB) often coincide with the monthly hormonal cycle and tend to subside after menopause. They can also be present for the whole month, but FB tissue will commonly increase and decrease in size and tenderness throughout the month. FB lumps are moveable when pressed and manipulated, as is opposed to cancerous lumps, which are fixed, or stuck, to the underlying tissue.

Root Causes

As the name would imply, there are fibrotic and cystic changes in the breast tissue. The most likely cause is that the cycle of estrogen and progesterone stimulate these changes. Hormonal imbalance, with estrogen dominance, is an important consideration.

Testing

- Fractionated Estrogens
- Progesterone
- Sex Hormone Binding Globulin
- CMP (primarily for liver function tests)

Other Considerations

A comprehensive hormone panel with urinary metabolites, and/or hormone cycle mapping, may be helpful in getting a deeper understanding of hormonal imbalance and how to treat.

Treatment

Treatment is focused on hormonal balancing, hormone detoxification, and avoiding common triggers.

Dietary Approach

- Avoid caffeine, including tea, and chocolate. Doing so is shown to improve symptoms in the majority of women.
- Get 30–50g fiber daily.
- Avoid processed and fast foods; focus on plants and whole foods.
- Decrease or eliminate alcohol.
- Eat Brassica family plants regularly.
- Avoid BPA. Discard all plastic water bottles and plastic food storage.

Herbs/Supplements

- N-Acetylcysteine – 600mg one to two times daily
- Selenium – 100mcg daily

Drink tea of these phytoestrogen plants often, either individually or in combination. Steep 1 tbsp of herb per cup of hot water for about 5 minutes. Licorice root needs to be decocted (simmered for 10–15 minutes) instead of steeped.

- Red Clover (*Trifolium pratense*)
- Calendula (*Calendula officinalis*)
- Plantain (*Plantago spp.*)
- Licorice (*Glycyrrhiza glabra*)

FIBROCYSTIC BREAST HERBAL TINCTURE FORMULA

Chaste Tree (*Vitex agnus-castus*)
Dong Quai (*Angelica sinensis*)
Dandelion Root (*Taraxacum officinale*)
Burdock (*Arctium lappa*)
Milk Thistle (*Silybum marianum*)
Red Root (*Ceanothus americanus*)

Mix 35% Chaste Tree, 30% Dong Quai, 15% Dandelion Root, 10% Burdock, 5% Milk Thistle, 5% Red Root. Take 2–4 droppersful two to three times daily

Lifestyle Changes

Diet and exercise are the most important areas to put energy into to improve hormone detoxification and facilitate a healthy hormonal cycle. Exercise of any kind is good, but work on producing a strong sweat at least two to three times a week. Weight training is especially effective.

Perform contrast hydrotherapy ahead of the onset of discomfort. Do this at least one to two times daily throughout the discomfort stage.

Affirmation

My feminine nature flows into all aspects of my life in a balanced and loving way.

FIBROIDS, UTERINE

Symptoms

- Abnormal uterine bleeding (i.e., heavy bleeding, prolonged bleeding)
- Pressure/discomfort/pain in pelvis
- Infertility
- Urinary frequency
- Constipation

Fibroids can also contribute to spontaneous abortion, abnormal fetal presentations, and increased postpartum hemorrhage.

Root Causes

These are benign uterine tumors of the smooth muscle of the uterine wall. Since they're benign, this means they aren't cancerous.

Fibroids are quite common, present in 70 percent of women by the age of 45. Exact cause is unknown, but evidence points toward genetic susceptibilities and largely lifestyle factors. Estrogen and progesterone, possibly when imbalanced, likely play roles in fibroid growth as well. Fibroid tissues can have increased receptors present for both of these hormones.

Known risk factors include:

- Alcohol (especially beer)
- Family history
- Early onset of menstruation
- Obesity
- Vitamin D deficiency
- Pro-inflammatory diet

Testing

- Fractionated estrogens
- Progesterone
- Sex hormone binding globulin
- CMP
- Vitamin D

- Pelvic exam
- Transvaginal ultrasound (US)

Other Considerations

A comprehensive hormone panel with urinary metabolites, and/or cycle mapping, may be helpful in getting a deeper understanding of hormonal imbalance and how to treat.

Treatment

Much of the treatment here, beyond foundational health components, is focused on balancing hormones and decreasing excess estrogen.

Dietary Approach

- Get 30–50g fiber daily.
- Avoid processed and fast foods; focus on plants and whole foods.
- Decrease or eliminate alcohol, especially beer.
- Eat Brassica family plants regularly.
- Avoid BPA. Discard all plastic water bottles and plastic food storage.

Herbs/Supplements

- N-Acetylcysteine – 600mg two to three times daily
- Selenium – 100mcg daily
- Vitamin D – 2000–5000IU daily

Drink tea of these phytoestrogen plants often, either individually or in combination. Steep 1 tbsp of herb per cup of hot water for about 5 minutes. Licorice root needs to be decocted instead of steeped.

- Red Clover (*Trifolium pratense*)
- Calendula (*Calendula officinalis*)
- Plantain (*Plantago spp.*)
- Licorice (*Glycyrrhiza glabra*)

HERBAL FIBROID TINCTURE FORMULA

Chaste Tree (*Vitex agnus-castus*)
Dong Quai (*Angelica sinensis*)

Burdock *(Arctium lappa)*
Dandelion Root *(Taraxacum officinale)*
Black Cohosh *(Actaea racemosa)*
Calendula *(Calendula officinalis)*
Red Root *(Ceanothus americanus)*

30% Chaste Tree, 25% Dong Quai, 15% Burdock, 10% Dandelion Root, 10% Black Cohosh, 5% Calendula, 5% Red Root. Take 2–4 droppersful two to three times daily.

Lifestyle Changes

Diet and exercise are the most important areas to put energy into in order to decrease any inflammation present and improve bodily detoxification.

Contrast hydrotherapy can improve circulation and lymph flow in the pelvis. Use the hydrotherapy method, being sure focusing on the pelvic region.

Affirmation

I let my emotions and thoughts flow through me like water in the river rock. I don't hold on.

FIBROMYALGIA

Symptoms

- Chronic musculoskeletal pain, often with tenderness of many areas of the body with pressure.
- Pain disproportionate to the stimulus
- Obvious reasons for the pain are typically absent

The pain in fibromyalgia (FM) is also generalized, as opposed to specific areas, and it typically doesn't need provocation to elicit it. It's more often an ever-present pain that waxes and wanes with activity and stress.

Besides pain, many other symptoms are common and can include:

- Fatigue
- Insomnia
- Depression and/or anxiety
- Headaches
- Irritable bowel syndrome
- Chest pain
- Shortness of breath
- Hypersensitivity to noise, smell, light, etc.
- Difficulty concentrating/brain fog

Root Causes

The cause of FM is not known. For this reason, many people suffer chronically. The pervading thought is that there is central sensitization. Essentially, this is when there is a heightened perception and sensitivity to pain because the brain is getting louder signals than it should, or sometimes when there doesn't need to be any pain signal at all.

There are many areas to look for potential causation, however. Nutrient deficiencies, gut dysbiosis, chronic infections, hormone imbalance, neurotransmitter imbalance, and toxic metals are all potential contributors that need to be considered. FM is more common with a history of trauma or post-traumatic stress disorder (PTSD).

FM is often triggered by a major stress to the body, mind, or emotions. Child-birth, viral infections like Lyme disease, operations, and death of a loved one are all possible triggers.

Testing

- CBC
- CMP
- hsCRP
- ESR
- TSH
- Lipid Panel
- Fractionated Estrogens
- Progesterone
- Testosterone
- Sex Hormone Binding Globulin
- Vitamin D
- Iron Panel with Ferritin
- RBC Magnesium
- RBC Folate

Other Considerations

- Food Elimination/ Re-Challenge Diet
- fT3, tT3, fT4, and tT4
- Comprehensive Stool Analysis
- Urine Toxic Metals Screen
- Epstein-Barr Virus Panel
- ANA w/reflex cascade
- Comprehensive nutrient panel
- Lyme Disease Panel and other tickborne illnesses
- Sinus Culture for Mold and Multiple Antibiotic Resistant Coagulase Negative Staphylococci (MARConS)
- Mold Toxins (Urine or Blood)

Treatment

Dietary Approach

- Eliminate food intolerances.
- Eat a high antioxidant and bioflavonoid-rich diet.
- Experiment with a vegetarian or vegan diet for at least six weeks each.
- Eat Brassica family plants regularly.
- Eat beets a couple of times a week.
- Get 30–50g fiber daily.
- Increase protein, at least 1–1.2g/kg body weight daily.

Herbs/Supplements

- N-Acetylcysteine – 600–900mg two to three times daily
- Vitamin A – 1500–3000mcg daily
- Vitamin C – 1g two to three times daily
- Vitamin E – 250mg daily
- Selenium – 100mcg daily
- Magnesium – 300–600mg daily at bedtime
- Vitamin B Complex – one serving daily
- Vitamin D – 2000–5000IU daily
- Full spectrum, organic, cannabidiol (CBD) extract – 10–20mg twice daily (there is research showing decreased endocannabinoids in FM patients)

FIBROMYALGIA HERBAL TINCTURE FORMULA

Siberian Ginseng (*Eleutherococcus senticosus*)
Schisandra (*Schisandra chinensis*)
Holy Basil, aka Tulsi (*Ocimum sanctum*)
Burdock (*Arctium lappa*)
Dandelion Root (*Taraxacum officinale*)
California Poppy (*Eschscholzia californica*)
Licorice Root (*Glycyrrhiza glabra*)

Mix 20% Siberian Ginseng, 15% Schisandra, 15% Holy Basil, 15% Burdock, 15% Dandelion Root, 15% California Poppy, 5% Licorice Root. Take 2–4 droppersful two to three times daily. Take two to three months before assessing effect.

Lifestyle Changes

Exercise plays a big role in recovery. As you implement the nutrients and herbs listed here, your body will be more able to move and for longer.

Sweat, in that same fashion, is also beneficial. Sweat for at least 20 minutes, at least three times a week in a sauna to start. A hot bath is a good substitute for a sauna, too. Doing so will help decrease total body burden of toxins.

Stop smoking to reduce the oxidative stress on the body.

Counseling and trauma therapy are important components in addressing FM.

Eye movement desensitization and reprocessing (EMDR), somatic therapy, and neurofeedback are a few additional therapies I highly recommend.

Many people with FM lose hope that improvement or resolution is possible. However, know that it's entirely possible. Remain positive about finding the right practitioners and therapeutics you need for your healing. You aren't out of options until you've given up searching.

Affirmation

Where there's a will, there's a way. I embrace my existence and the lessons to be learned and commit to finding my healing path.

HASHIMOTO'S THYROIDITIS

Symptoms

- Fatigue
- Constipation
- Weight gain

- Cold intolerance
- Dry skin

As Hashimoto thyroiditis (HT) advances, symptoms can include:

- Hair loss
- Depression
- Decreased sweating
- Dementia
- Joint/muscle pain

- Sleep apnea
- Menstrual cycle irregularities
- Peripheral neuropathy
- Goiter
- Decreased deep tendon reflexes

Onset of HT is commonly slow to progress, typically over a span of years.

Root Causes

HT is an autoimmune (AI) condition. It's the most common cause of hypothyroidism in the United States. In HT, the immune system makes antibodies that trigger the immune system to attack the thyroid gland. As this destruction happens, there's less thyroid gland available to make thyroid hormone, and hypothyroidism ensues, slowly worsening over time.

AI illness is inflammatory in nature, and is often associated with traumatic, emotional, and physical events, viral infections, leaky gut, gut dysbiosis, and in the case of HT, it also has correlation with celiac disease.

Testing

- TSH
- fT3, tT3, tT4 and fT4
- Thyroid Peroxidase Antibody (Anti-TPO)
- Thyroglobulin Antibody (Anti-Tg)

- CBC
- CMP
- Lipid Panel
- CRP

Other Considerations

- Celiac disease
- Thyroid Ultrasound if nodules are suspected
- Food Elimination/Re-Challenge to assess for intolerances/sensitivities
- Epstein-Barr Virus Panel to assess for potential reactivation

Treatment

The treatment for HT should never just be thyroid hormone replacement alone. Although it's important, addressing the underlying inflammation and immune system dysregulation is key.

Dietary Approach

- Follow an anti-inflammatory diet, with 7–10 servings of vegetables daily.
- Identify and eliminate food intolerances.
- Avoid fast food and processed foods.
- Eat as clean as possible, using the Dirty Dozen by the EWG as a starting point.

It's also worth considering eliminating gluten for at least a six- to 12-month period and re-assessing disease activity.

Herbs/Supplements

- Broad Spectrum Probiotic daily
- N-Acetylcysteine – 600mg one to two times daily
- Selenium – 100mcg daily
- Vitamin C – 1000mg two to three times daily
- Vitamin E – 250mg daily
- Vitamin D – 2000–5000IU daily
- Fish Oil – 1–2g daily
- Curcumin – 2g daily

HASHIMOTO'S THYROIDITIS HERBAL TINCTURE FORMULA

Siberian Ginseng (*Eleutherococcus senticosus*)
Astragalus (*Astragalus membranaceus*)
Devil's Club (*Oplopanax horridus*)

Rhodiola (*Rhodiola rosea*)
Licorice (*Glycyrrhiza glabra*)

Mix 25% Siberian Ginseng, 25% Astragalus, 25% Devil's Club, 20% Rhodiola, 5% Licorice. Take 2–4 droppersful two to three times daily.

Lifestyle Changes

Focus energy on improving quality and quantity of sleep and stress management. See the insomnia section (page 140) if this is a major problem. Aim for seven to eight hours of uninterrupted sleep each night. Go to bed by 11 p.m.

As with any AI condition, stress management and reduction practices, such as meditation and/or yoga, are necessary in order for the immune system to regain balance. Chronic stress takes a toll on the adrenal glands as well and can create additional fatigue beyond hypothyroidism. Find what works for you to decompress and center yourself, and commit to it regularly.

Affirmation

I show up in my life passionately and authentically. I am unafraid to show my true self and beliefs.

HEADACHES & MIGRAINES

Symptoms

Tension headache symptoms include:

- Generalized pain
- Typically more mild than migraines
- Tight neck and shoulders

Migraine headache symptoms include:

- Pain anywhere in the head, often one-sided, sometimes including the face
- Character of pain can vary (throbbing, shooting, pressing, etc.)
- Sensitivity to light, sound, smell, etc.
- Nausea/vomiting
- Aura before and/or after

Depending on the type of headache, symptoms can last from less than an hour to multiple days. Likewise, the severity of symptoms can also be mild to debilitating.

Root Causes

Tension headaches are caused by muscular and fascial tension, oftentimes from a distant location, like the shoulders and neck. The tension gets translated to the fascia and muscles of the scalp and head. This tension itself creates pain, but can also trap nerves and blood vessels, creating pain from these routes.

Various nervous system and vascular affects in the brain and head cause migraine headaches. There is overexcitability in portions of the nervous system, and there are changes in blood flow as well as inflammation of arteries of the head and the dura mater of the brain. Migraines can have a wide variety of triggers, including foods, alcohol (especially wine), all manner of chemicals, bright light, weather and barometric changes, sleep disturbance, hormones, and hypoglycemia.

Stress also plays a big role in headaches. It's quite common for individuals with chronic headaches to be able to use the frequency of headache symptoms as a gauge for how stressed they've been.

Trigger points in other muscles like the scalene and trapezius can also cause headaches.

Testing

Testing is to rule out other conditions where headache is a secondary symptom or uncover contributing factors. Headache diagnosis is otherwise based on symptoms.

- CBC
- CMP
- Sex Hormone Panel
- CRP
- HbA1C
- RBC Magnesium
- Food Elimination/Re-Challenge to assess for intolerances/sensitivities

Treatment

Dietary Approach

Migraines:

- Avoid red wine/other sulfite-containing foods.
- Eliminate coffee for a month as a test.
- Eliminate food intolerances.

Tension Headaches:

- Increase magnesium-rich foods.
- Eat 7–10 servings of a variety of vegetables daily to ensure adequate mineral intake.

Herbs/Supplements

Migraine Headache:

- Magnesium – 300–600mg daily
- Vitamin B Complex – one serving daily
- Melatonin – 3mg 30 minutes before bed as a prophylaxis trial
- N-Acetylcysteine – 600mg one to two times daily

MIGRAINE HERBAL TINCTURE FORMULA (PREVENTIVE)

Milky Oats (*Avena sativa*)
Passionflower (*Passiflora incarnata*)
Betony (*Stachys officinalis*)
Turmeric (*Curcuma longa*)
Licorice (*Glycyrrhiza glabra*)
Dandelion Root (*Taraxacum officinale*)

Mix 20% Milky Oats, 20% Passionflower, 20% Betony, 20% Turmeric, 10% Licorice, 10% Dandelion Root. Take 2–4 droppersful two to three times daily.

Tension Headache:

- Magnesium – 150–300mg twice daily

TENSION HEADACHE HERBAL TINCTURE FORMULA (ACUTE/DURING HEADACHE)

Cramp Bark (*Viburnum opulus*)
California Poppy (*Eschscholzia californica*)
Skullcap (*Scutellaria lateriflora*)
Passionflower (*Passiflora incarnata*)
Kava Kava (*Piper methysticum*)
Valerian (*Valeriana officinalis*)

Mix 20% Cramp Bark, 20% California Poppy, 15% Skullcap, 15% Passionflower, 15% Kava Kava, 15% Valerian. Take 2–5 droppersful three to four times daily, depending on headache severity. This formula may be sedative in nature to sensitive individuals.

Lifestyle Changes

Sleep disturbance is a major trigger for headaches. If you have sleep problems of any kind, addressing these appropriately will likely decrease frequency of headaches. Sleep apnea and insomnia in particular should be addressed.

Start a daily mindfulness meditation practice. With increased body awareness, you can sometimes stop a headache before it becomes a problem.

Neurofeedback and biofeedback are both strongly recommended for migraine treatment.

For tension headaches, progressive muscle relaxation is a specific technique that is often beneficial.

Soma, Rolfing, or other types of fascial work and neuromuscular reintegration techniques work well and can resolve recurrent tension headaches.

Lastly, perineural injection therapy (PIT) and trigger point injections are a treatment to consider for any type of headache.

Affirmation

I actively address and change the things that don't bring me joy and peace in my life.

HEART DISEASE

Symptoms

Heart disease, a term that's interchangeable with cardiovascular disease (CVD), isn't a single thing. It encompasses a variety of conditions, such as congestive heart failure (CHF), atherosclerosis, and arrhythmias. CVD symptoms are primarily due to changes in the circulation. The electrical conduction system of the heart can also be affected in CVD. The symptoms are too numerous to list, but the most common areas affected will be the heart itself, the lungs, the kidneys, and any area where there is decreased circulation and oxygenation.

Root Causes

The most common causes of the most common type of CVD, atherosclerosis, is inflammation due to modern lifestyle, diet and environmental toxin exposures. Chronic inflammation and hypertension damages the walls of blood vessels. The body uses cholesterol like a bandage to cover that spot of inflammation and damage. With continued damage and inflammation, the plaques harden and get calcified. This process can then lead to stroke and heart attack. Note that the cholesterol is *not* the problem; the inflammation and hypertension are. The cholesterol is doing an important job.

Heart valve problems lead to decreased outflow from the heart, congestive heart failure, and lung problems. Issues of heart valves can be caused by infections, aging, and can be congenital as well.

Cardiomyopathy is a heart condition that can be caused by infections and drug toxicity.

Arrhythmias are fairly common and can be the result of different mineral deficiencies, stress, and inborn errors in electrical conduction.

It's also possible to get infections in different parts of the heart, with both viruses and bacteria.

Testing

- CBC
- CMP
- Lipid Panel
- hsCRP

- Hemoglobin A1C
- Homocysteine
- Uric Acid
- TSH

Other Considerations

- Coronary Calcium Score (atherosclerosis)
- Echocardiogram (valves or congestive heart failure)
- EKG (palpitations and arrhythmias)
- Cardiac Stress Test
- There are also large specialized cardiovascular risk panels available through many labs.

There are numerous tests for specific conditions. The blood labs listed here will give a basic window into areas to assess for other conditions to be addressed, such as diabetes and fatty liver.

Treatment

The treatments here are focused primarily on atherosclerosis and its negative effects, because it causes the most CVD. Preventing and reversing atherosclerosis isn't all that complicated. It takes a commitment to healthy diet and lifestyle change, however. To heal the cardiovascular system from atherosclerosis, maintaining a healthy diet, lifestyle, body weight, and blood sugar control are not just ideas to consider—they are required.

Dietary Approach

No one diet is perfect for everyone. Vegetarian, vegan, and Mediterranean diets are different variations of a whole-food, plant-based diet that can be effective in treating and preventing CVD. If you're eating variety, clean, whole foods, and plant-based, the name of the diet and its details probably don't matter much. It's most important to remove and replace inflammatory food and beverage choices.

- Eliminate sugar, processed, and fast foods.
- Eat organic, at least the Dirty Dozen by the EWG and wheat.
- Avoid industrial seed/vegetable oils (i.e., corn, soy, cottonseed, etc.).
- Eat 1–2 servings dark berries daily.
- Eat 1–2 fresh cloves of garlic daily. Adding fresh garlic at the end of cooking is best.

Herbs/Supplements

ATHEROSCLEROSIS

- Selenium – 100mcg daily
- N-Acetylcysteine – 600mg two to three times daily
- Vitamin C – 1g two to three times daily
- Vitamin E – 250mg daily
- Fish Oil – 1–2g daily
- Vitamin K2 – 45mcg daily
- Hawthorne (*Crataegus oxyacantha*) leaf, flower, and berry extract – 1–2g daily
- Hawthorne Berry Solid Extract – ⅛ tsp twice daily
- Curcumin – 1–2g daily

ARRHYTHMIA

Depending on the arrhythmia, different minerals can contribute to improvement. Try a multimineral to start and see whether there is improvement. Hawthorne can also help arrhythmias.

Lifestyle Changes

Regular exercise and addressing sleep issues, in particular sleep apnea, are necessary to improve CVD. Sleep apnea causes a great deal of inflammation in the body. Losing weight and the therapies list here will help with apnea, but a CPAP is necessary until apnea is resolved.

Heart rate variability training can be used to treat hypertension, arrhythmias, and is one of the best therapies someone can do after a heart attack to prevent recurrence.

Affirmation

I tend to my heart and am open to experiencing, joy, fun, and love.

HEARTBURN & GASTROESOPHAGEAL REFLUX DISEASE (GERD)

Symptoms

- Burning chest pain
- Sore throat (from acid)
- Wheezing, cough, or hoarseness from aspiration of acid
- Rising of food and acid into mouth

Heartburn itself is a symptom caused by GERD. Long-term acid reflux leads to inflammation of the esophagus and cellular changes, which increase the risk for esophageal cancer. Lung damage can also be present from chronic aspiration, which oftentimes occurs while sleeping.

Root Causes

GERD is caused by a relaxation of the muscular junction where the esophagus meets the stomach. This junction is called the lower esophageal sphincter (LES). LES is essentially a one-way muscle, and if it relaxes, the pressure present on the stomach (from the abdomen contents) outweighs the pressure above, and reflux of the stomach contents results. Heartburn can be periodic as well. In these cases, it happens from particular aggravations, versus GERD, which happens on a chronic basis.

Stomach acid is a trigger for the LES to stay closed. If there is *too little acid*, this can cause reflux. There are also foods that commonly trigger reflux and are assumed to relax the LES, which include chocolate, peppermint, coffee, garlic, and onions. On the other hand, too much stomach acid can also cause heartburn symptoms. However, with the LES functioning properly, there should be less concern of this. H. pylori is a bacterium that can be present chronically in the stomach and sometimes causes too little or too much acid production.

An atonic, or weak, LES will cause GERD, as well as some anatomical conditions, like hiatal hernia.

Alcohol, tobacco, obesity, and various medications, such as anticholinergics, antihistamines, tricyclic antidepressants, calcium channel blockers, progesterone, and nitrates, are all risk factors for reflux.

Testing

- CMP
- Celiac Disease Panel
- Vitamin D
- Food Elimination/Re-Challenge to assess for intolerances/sensitivities

If an ulcer and bleeding is suspected:

- Ferritin
- CBC
- Fecal Occult Blood

Imaging to Consider:

- Endoscopy with biopsy for H. pylori
- Ultrasound if a mass is suspected

Other Considerations

- H. pylori Stool Antigen
- Heidelberg Test
- Comprehensive Stool Analysis and Infection Screen (screen for a wide range of bacteria, viruses, and parasites)

Treatment

Dietary Approach

Start by decreasing, or avoiding all together, the foods that appear to relax the LES: chocolate, coffee, alcohol, and peppermint. Peppermint can also be beneficial for heartburn and reflux because of its other gastrointestinal effects. Experimentation is probably the best here. Also, some people will avoid onions and garlic for heartburn. Unless you clearly notice they are problems for you, keep them in your diet, as they have a great deal of health benefits.

- Avoid fried/processed foods.
- Eliminate known or suspected food intolerances.
- Stop eating three hours before bed.
- Be mindful of chewing food completely.

Herbs/Supplements

- Digestive Enzyme – one serving size with primary meals
- Digestive Bitters – 5–10 drops on the back of the tongue, 5–15 minutes before meals, or three times daily
- Demulcent herb preparation (Slippery Elm or Marshmallow Root) – drink two to three times daily, *do not take at the same time as medications and supplements as they can decrease absorption*
- Deglycyrrhizinated Licorice (DGL) – one chewable tablet two to three times daily
- Broad Spectrum Probiotic Daily
- Tea of Lemon Balm *(Melissa officinalis)*, Chamomile *(Matricaria recutita)*, and/or Fennel Seed *(Foeniculum vulgare)* – 1 tbsp per cup water two to three times daily. Chamomile and Lemon Balm can steep for 5 minutes. Fennel needs to be decocted for 10–15 minutes with a lid on the pot.

REFLUX HERBAL TINCTURE FORMULA (PREVENTIVE)

Turmeric *(Curcuma longa)*
Dandelion Root *(Taraxacum officinale)*
Fennel Seed *(Foeniculum vulgare)*
Lemon Balm *(Melissa officinalis)*
Chamomile *(Matricaria recutita)*

Mix 25% Turmeric, 25% Dandelion Root, 20% Fennel Seed, 15% Lemon Balm, 15% Chamomile. Take 2–4 droppersful two to three times daily.

Lifestyle Changes

Stress reduction and appropriate management can play a profound role for some people in relieving reflux and heartburn. Exercise, daily mindfulness meditation practice, and simply taking time for quiet and reflection daily are all possible stress modifying behaviors.

Try sleeping reclined while working on healing GERD and heartburn.

Visceral manipulation is a specialized form of hands-on therapy and is a gentle method to assist with heartburn and GERD.

Affirmation

I breathe with ease and release my fears and anxieties around my life.

HEAVY METAL TOXICITY

Symptoms

Common symptoms that may present are:

- Brain fog/confusion
- Headache
- Nausea/vomiting
- Fatigue
- Depression and/or anxiety
- Irritability
- Fevers
- Neuropathies
- Muscle, abdominal, or nerve pains
- All manner of behavioral changes

Symptoms depend on the type of metal present, the level and frequency of exposure, and the tissue in which it accumulates in the body. Typical symptoms are somewhat nonspecific, and nearly any body system can be affected.

Root Causes

Heavy metals occur naturally in the soil and in different amounts in water supplies. Aside from these exposures, heavy metals are consistently present in different foods, herbs, and even in things like children's toys manufactured on an industrial scale.

When foods are grown in soils with high heavy metal contents, some of it ends up in the food. Pesticides and herbicides are other contributors to heavy metals in our food system and the environment. Some heavy metals are used in various industries and then end up in our environment, such as mercury, which ends up in water, and then in fish, which we then accumulate in large amounts in our body from eating those fish.

Although our bodies can excrete heavy metals and some metals are used in our bodies for important purposes, if we take in more than we can excrete, we start to bioaccumulate and negative effects can ensue.

Testing

Testing should be done to both rule out other conditions and to understand the biologic effects of heavy metal toxicity on a person if toxicity is known to be present.

- Urine Toxic Metals Screen (Unprovoked); Provoked can be done afterward if it's highly suspected to see how much gets released, but if it's elevated on unprovoked testing there's really no need.
- CBC
- CMP
- CRP
- TSH
- Ferritin
- RBC Magnesium
- Zinc
- Copper
- Ceruloplasmin

Treatment

The three main goals with treatment are to eliminate exposure, promote excretion, and support the negatively affected body systems to heal.

Dietary Approach

With regard to heavy metal toxicity, the focus needs to be on eating clean and a lot of plants. Eat organic and low-metal burden foods. Doing so requires some research. Arsenic is high in rice, for example. If you eat fish, learn what fish are lowest in mercury. Understand the primary food, water, and medicine exposures for the metal(s) you have tested high for. In addition, ensure adequate fiber at 30–50g daily and 7–10 servings of vegetables daily. This ensures bile, which carries toxins from the liver, is bound up and excreted.

Herbs/Supplements

- Vitamin C – 1g two to three times daily
- Vitamin E – 250mcg daily
- N-Acetylcysteine – 600mg two to three times daily
- Selenium – 100mcg daily

- Multimineral – one serving daily
- Vitamin B Complex – one serving daily
- CoQ10 – 100–200mg daily

LIVER DETOX SUPPORT HERBAL TINCTURE FORMULA

Turmeric (*Curcuma longa*)
Dandelion Root (*Taraxacum officinale*)
Burdock (*Arctium lappa*)
Milk Thistle (*Silybum marianum*)
Licorice (*Glycyrrhiza glabra*)

Mix 25% Turmeric, 25% Dandelion Root, 20% Burdock, 20% Milk Thistle, 10% Licorice. Take 2–4 droppersful two to three times daily long term.

Lifestyle Changes

Detox requires the support of healthy sleep and consistent exercise. If insomnia is an issue, see the treatment options on page 140.

Sweating is one of the most effective therapeutics for heavy metal toxicity. Sweat for at least 20 minutes daily, three times weekly, indefinitely. The sauna is the easiest venue for sweating long term.

Review your water quality reports. Doing so is especially important if you're drinking from a well, as some regions have naturally high metal levels due to their geology.

Affirmation

I release that which does not serve me and harms me. I continually fill myself up with new experience and vitality.

HYPERTENSION

Symptoms

Consistent blood pressure (BP) elevation of:

- Systolic (top number) over 130

and/or

- Diastolic (bottom number) is above 80

Hypertension (HT), or elevated BP, is itself a symptom. There usually aren't other symptoms involved with HT, unless the BP is extremely elevated, at which point symptoms like headache and tinnitus (ringing in ears) can take place.

The long-term sequelae of untreated HT are primarily cardiovascular and kidney disease.

Root Causes

BP is controlled by various factors, such as how much fluid is in the system, how hard and fast the heart beats, and how much resistance is present at the end of the arteries in the periphery.

HT is usually primary, meaning not caused by another condition. In this scenario, there are usually a collection of variables that are involved in the resultant symptom of HT. Genetics can play a role in the cause by increasing the susceptibility of an individual to get HT from certain environmental factors. Some factors commonly associated with HT are an inflammatory diet, or standard American diet (SAD), high sodium intake, diabetes, and obesity. Stress and strong emotions can cause elevated BP in the moment, but when experienced chronically, they directly contribute to HT for many people.

Common secondary causes are a variety of kidney conditions, primary aldosteronism and obstructive sleep apnea. Lead is a well-established environmental cause of HT.

Testing

- CBC
- CMP
- Lipid Panel
- TSH

- hsCRP
- Uric Acid
- Homocysteine
- UA, Dipstick

Other Considerations

Consider secondary causes if the diagnosis is essential HT, the BP isn't improving with diet and lifestyle, and especially if the HT takes multiple medications to improve. Plasma Renin Activity (PRA) is a test for primary hyperaldosteronism. Heavy metal, or specifically lead testing, is another consideration in treating resistant HT.

Treatment

Dietary Approach

A plant-based diet with a wide variety of vegetables and fruits is imperative in treating HT. If adhered to on a regular basis, the dietary constructs laid out in chapter 2 will likely be beneficial. These are the basic tenets of whole food, plant-based, clean, and variety eating. There are also various, more specific diets that may be useful to follow, including the Mediterranean diet, dietary approaches to stop hypertension (DASH) diet, and vegetarian.

- Eat foods high in magnesium.
- Eat foods high in potassium.
- Eat foods high in calcium.
- Some people respond well to sodium reduction. 6g or less of salt is a therapeutic reduction, but can also be challenging.
- Reduce alcohol consumption.
- Eat 1–2 servings dark berries daily.
- Eat dark chocolate regularly with little to no sugar added.
- Eliminate sugar.
- Processed and fast foods need to be avoided.
- Avoid industrial seed/vegetable oils (i.e., corn, soy, cottonseed, etc.).
- Eat 7–10 servings of vegetables daily.
- Get 30–50g fiber daily.

Herbs/Supplements

- Magnesium – 150–300mg twice daily
- Vitamin C – 1g two to three times daily
- Vitamin B Complex – one serving daily
- Hawthorne *(Crataegus spp.)* Extract with berry, leaf, and flower – 500mg two to four times daily for at least three to nine months

Lifestyle Changes

Although supplementation can help with HT, lifestyle factors will likely provide the most profound and lasting results. Exercise should include a combination of weight training and cardio. Incorporating yoga or tai chi is another way to get movement and also reduce stress.

Smoking is inflammatory and contributes to HT. Put a cessation plan in place. Counseling and hypnosis can be helpful with quitting smoking.

Sleep apnea is a serious condition that increases all-cause mortality. If you snore or stop breathing in your sleep, get a referral to a sleep specialist for appropriate testing and treatment.

Heart rate variability (HRV) training and mindfulness training are two practices that directly and positively impact HT.

Affirmation

I live my day with ease, breathing into my emotions, letting stress roll off me like water off a duck's back.

HYPOTHYROIDISM

Symptoms

- Fatigue
- Constipation
- Weight gain
- Cold intolerance
- Dry skin
- Hair loss
- Depression
- Decreased sweating
- Dementia
- Joint/muscle pain
- Sleep apnea
- Menstrual cycle irregularities
- Peripheral neuropathy
- Swelling around eyes
- Slow heart rate
- Hoarse voice
- Goiter
- Decreased deep tendon reflexes

These are just some of the possible hypothyroidism symptoms. Symptoms are those consistent with decreased metabolic functions.

Root Causes

Hypothyroidism means having too little thyroid hormone present for healthy function. Hashimoto's thyroiditis, an autoimmune condition, is the most common cause of hypothyroidism in the United States. If not immune mediated, frank hypothyroidism is most typically caused by radiation or surgery to the thyroid, medications, or iodine deficiency.

Although not near as drastic as full-fledged hypothyroidism, the thyroid gland can also simply underfunction and cause symptoms as well. The thyroid is a relatively sensitive organ to environmental stressors, such as infections and toxins of various sorts. It's common in clinical practice to see individuals, usually women, with an underfunctioning thyroid gland that is secondary to other imbalances.

These conditions may be due to lifestyle, chronic inflammation, or adrenal fatigue/burnout.

It's possible for the thyroid gland to make enough T4 thyroid hormone but not adequately convert it to T3, which is the active thyroid hormone in the body. This scenario appears to be in response to inflammation and various chronic illnesses.

Testing

- TSH
- fT3, tT3, fT4, and tT4
- Thyroid Peroxidase Antibody (Anti-TPO)
- Thyroglobulin Antibody (Anti-Tg)
- CBC
- CMP
- hsCRP

Other Considerations

- 24-hour Urine Iodine Excretion
- 24-hour Urine Cortisol, which maps the cycle as well as the total
- Thyroid Ultrasound if nodules are suspected
- Food Elimination/Re-Challenge to assess for intolerances/sensitivities

Treatment

Dietary Approach

A plant-based diet that is as toxin-free as possible sets the stage for success here. Having adequate fiber is also necessary to aid in consistent detoxification.

- Avoid any known food intolerances.
- Eliminate sugar.
- Reduce caffeine to 1–2 servings of coffee daily.
- Eat organic, at least the Dirty Dozen by the EWG as well as wheat and oats.
- Eat 7–10 servings of vegetables daily.
- Get 30–50g fiber daily.
- Eat beets weekly.
- Eat copious amounts of onions and garlic.

Herbs/Supplements

- Selenium – 100mcg daily
- N-Acetylcysteine – 600mg two to three times daily
- Vitamin A – 1500–3000mcg daily
- Vitamin C – 1g two to three times daily
- Vitamin E – 250mg daily
- L-tyrosine – 500mg daily
- Vitamin B Complex – one serving daily
- Zinc* – 15mg daily

HYPOTHYROIDISM HERBAL TINCTURE FORMULA 1

Rhodiola (*Rhodiola rosea*)
Siberian Ginseng (*Eleutherococcus senticosus*)
Astragalus (*Astragalus membranaceus*)
Licorice (*Glycyrrhiza glabra*)

Mix 30% Rhodiola, 30% Siberian Ginseng, 30% Astragalus, 10% Licorice. Take 2–4 droppersful two to three times daily.

HYPOTHYROIDISM HERBAL TINCTURE FORMULA 2

Milk Thistle (*Silybum marianum*)
Schisandra (*Schisandra chinensis*)
Dandelion Leaf (*Taraxacum officinale*)
Holy Basil, aka Tulsi (*Ocimum sanctum*)

Mix equal parts Milk Thistle, Schisandra, Dandelion Leaf, and Holy Basil. Take 2–4 droppersful two to three time daily.

Lifestyle Changes

Going to bed by 11 p.m. and getting seven to eight hours of sleep is ideal. Your body needs this time to heal and repair.

With long-term zinc supplementation, you have to also supplement with 1–3mg/day of copper to avoid zinc-induced copper deficiency.

A little bit of exercise can go a long way. It can be hard when you are fatigued, but once you implement the dietary, herbal, and supplement protocols, your ability to exercise will increase. Start wherever you're at, maybe with simply walking. Continually push the edge of comfort though, so that your body adapts and your metabolism strengthens.

Affirmation

I show up in my life passionately and authentically. I am unafraid to show my true self and beliefs.

INFECTIONS

Symptoms

- Fever
- Body aches
- Fatigue

These are the most common symptoms, but many others are possible. Most symptoms related to infections depend on the infectious agent (i.e., bacteria, virus, parasite) and the body systems it invades (i.e., gut, lungs, sinuses).

Root Causes

Acute infections will, by definition, resolve on their own. When an infection doesn't get resolved and remains in the body chronically, there are a couple of main reasons: low immune function and/or a "stealthy" infectious agent.

Many organisms are able to evade the immune system and stay in the body permanently. Herpes simplex is an example of this. As long as the immune system stays relatively strong, they stay dormant for most people, at least the majority of the time. Some reasons for low immune function are poorly managed diabetes, chronic unmanaged stress, nutrient deficiencies, and chronic inflammation (whether from other health conditions or poor diet and lifestyle), and some chronic infections themselves can impact immune function. In addition, environmental toxins such as heavy metals and pesticides decrease immune function, along with various medications. There are also genetic disorders of the immune system that manifest as ineffective function.

Testing

- CBC
- CMP, Fasting
- CRP
- Neutrophil/Lymphocyte Ratio
- Hemoglobin A1C

Immune System-Specific Considerations:

- Serum IgG, IgA, IgE, IgM
- Compliment Levels

Chronic Infection Considerations:

- Epstein-Barr Virus Panel
- Cytomegalovirus
- Lyme Disease and other tickborne illnesses
- HIV
- Hepatitis C
- Sexually Transmitted Infections
- Intestinal Parasites
- Comprehensive Stool Pathogen Analysis

Treatment

The treatment approaches here will focus on immune stimulation and immune modulation (balancing), and foundational factors that support a healthy immune system.

Dietary Approach

It's not realistic to expect a healthy, functioning immune system without having a nutrient-dense, whole-food diet.

- Avoid inflammatory foods, like fast food and processed foods.
- Avoid known food intolerances.
- Eat 7–10 servings of vegetables daily.
- Follow the other dietary approaches in the diabetes section (page 80) for blood sugar control to minimize the negative immune system effects of blood sugar dysregulation.
- Eat a high bioflavonoid content daily.

Herbs/Supplements

ACUTE INFECTION

- Vitamin A – 2500–5000IU daily
- Vitamin E – 250mg daily

- Vitamin C – 1–2g daily
- Selenium – 100mcg daily
- Zinc – 15mg daily
- Broad Spectrum Probiotic – daily
- Vitamin D – 2000–5000IU daily

Stop after symptoms resolve. In treating a chronic infection, the supplement protocol in the Epstein-Barr and other viral infections section page 90 is the best approach.

IMMUNE MODULATING HERBAL TINCTURE FORMULA (CHRONIC INFECTIONS)

Astragalus (*Astragalus membranaceus*)
Siberian Ginseng (*Eleutherococcus senticosus*)
Devil's Club (*Oplopanax horridus*)
Ashwagandha (*Withania somnifera*)
Licorice (*Glycyrrhiza glabra*)

Mix 25% Astragalus, 25% Siberian Ginseng, 20% Devil's Club, 20% Ashwagandha, 10% Licorice. Take 2–4 droppersful two to three times daily.

This tincture is meant to be taken for at least three to six months for a weakened immune system and chronic infections.

ACUTE BACTERIAL INFECTION HERBAL TINCTURE FORMULA

Echinacea (*Echinacea spp.*)
Osha Root (*Ligusticum porteri*)
Oregon Grape (*Mahonia spp.*)
Licorice (*Glycyrrhiza glabra*)

Mix 30% Echinacea, 30% Osha, 20% Oregon Grape, 20% Licorice. Take 3–5 droppersful three to four times daily for three to five days.

ACUTE VIRAL INFECTION HERBAL TINCTURE FORMULA

Astragalus (*Astragalus membranaceus*)
Lomatium (*Lomatium dissectum*)*

Lomatium has been known to cause an itchy rash that can present over the whole body. Although I haven't seen this in practice with much use, it is a real phenomenon to be aware of. The rash ceases after stopping lomatium.

Olive Leaf (*Olea europaea*)
Licorice (*Glycyrrhiza glabra*) *

40% Astragalus, 20% Lomatium, 20% Olive Leaf, 20% Licorice. Take 3–5 droppersful three to four times daily for three to five days.

Lifestyle Changes

Much like what was said about diet, without healthy sleep, exercise, and other foundational health components, such as stress reduction and management, healthy immune function can't be expected. Get enough sleep and be sure to move your body on a regular basis. Pushing your body to adapt to exercise creates greater overall resiliency.

Tobacco use, in particular smoking, is very inflammatory. Quitting will improve immune function and overall health and vitality.

Affirmation

I am resilient in body, mind, and emotions.

---

*This much licorice could create elevated blood pressure in some, or worsen it in those who already have hypertension. The percent can be decreased to 5–10% if this is the case. The potential hypertensive effects will go away after licorice is stopped.

INFERTILITY

Symptoms

Infertility is the inability to conceive, or on repeated attempts there is a failure for conception to take place.

Root Causes

Infertility can happen for many different reasons, and it's a mistake not to assess both partners to understand where the problems are arising. Clinically speaking, both partners should always be assessed appropriately from the start.

In men, various defects in the sperm can create the problem. This is the cause in more than 35 percent of infertility cases. If the sperm can't get to their destination correctly or there aren't enough of them, the woman's level of fertility won't make a difference.

For women, problems with infertility can happen from a decrease in or simply no ovulation taking place. Low egg reserve is another possibility. There can also be problems in the shape of the Fallopian tubes or lesions present in them that can impair sperm motility and effective travel of the egg. In a small percentage of women, the cervical mucus is not of a consistency to facilitate penetration by sperm and sperm survival.

A variety of health factors can play a role in sperm health for men and in the various factors affecting a woman's fertility. Luckily, there is a lot to be done naturally.

Some factors that affect fertility in males and females are:

- Environmental toxins (BPA, pesticides, etc.)
- Inflammatory diets and processed foods
- Nutrient deficiencies
- Obesity
- Metabolic syndrome/diabetes

Polycystic ovary syndrome (PCOS) is one of the most common causes of infertility in the United States and is covered in its own section (page 165).

Testing

Men

- Sperm Analysis
- Testosterone (T)
- Follicle Stimulating Hormone (FSH)
- If low T, test Luteinizing Hormone (LH) and Prolactin
- Hemoglobin A1C
- CMP
- CBC

Women

- CMP
- CBC
- CRP
- Neutrophil/Lymphocyte Ratio (NLR)
- Lipid Panel
- Fractionated Estrogen
- Progesterone (Measured one week before the menstrual cycle can tell whether ovulation has happened.)
- Testosterone
- SHBG
- LH
- FSH
- Hormone Cycle Mapping and 24-Hour Urine Hormones and Metabolites
- Anti-Müllerian Hormone (AMH) Level and Antral Follicle Count (AFC) to test ovarian reserves
- Hysterosalpingography (specialized x-ray of uterus and Fallopian tubes)
- Pelvic Ultrasound to look at ovary size in the late follicular phase or other anatomical abnormalities

Other Considerations

If in vitro is being considered, explore testing for:

- Sperm Antibody Test
- Hypo-osmotic Swelling Test

- Hemizona and Sperm Penetration Assay
- Genetic Testing if there are very low or no sperm present

Treatment

Although reproduction is the most fundamental and critical aspect to not only humankind but also to all biological organisms, it's a sensitive system. In particular, the hormonal and reproductive systems are affected negatively by man-made chemicals and modern diets, which are pro-inflammatory and contain many toxins.

It's crucial that the foundational components of health come to the forefront of the effort to improve fertility. Just as both partners need to be assessed for issues leading to infertility, relationally speaking, both partners should bear the responsibility of improving diet, lifestyle factors, etc. to improve the chances of conception.

Dietary Approach

- Implement a plant-based, anti-inflammatory diet.
- Start eating as clean from toxins as possible.
- Eliminate refined sugar.
- Eat *at least* 1 cup beans or lentils daily.
- Eat 7–10 servings of vegetables daily.
- Eat small meals more frequently.
- Consume 30–50g fiber daily.
- Avoid processed and fast foods.
- Decrease or eliminate alcohol altogether.
- Avoid BPA. Discard all plastic water bottles and food storage.
- Decrease caffeine to 1–2 servings of coffee daily.
- Eat organic, at least the Dirty Dozen foods listed by the EWG, wheat, and oats.

Herbs/Supplements

MEN

- CoQ10 – 150mg twice daily
- L-Carnitine – 500mg twice daily
- Vitamin A – 1500–3000mcg daily

- Vitamin E – 250mg daily
- Vitamin C – 1g two to three times daily
- Selenium – 100mcg daily
- Zinc* – 15mg daily
- N-Acetyl Cysteine – 600–900mg two to three times daily
- Vitamin B Complex – one serving daily

WOMEN

- Quality Prenatal Vitamin
- N-Acetyl Cysteine – 600mg two times daily

Lifestyle Changes

Optimal sleep health is the most beneficial lifestyle change. Getting seven to eight hours of sleep each night is best.

Get exercise based on CDC guidelines, if possible. However, any movement and decrease in stagnancy is helpful.

Be gentle with yourself. Let go of any blame for infertility. Make self-care your priority. Patience is so important: Slow down and work toward seeing results in one year versus waiting just a few months.

Be intimate for the sake of intimacy. Sex can start to feel like a job for couples trying to conceive. Do you have sex or other intimacy outside of the short window of ovulation every month? Bring more of this activity in. In that same vein, counseling for both individuals and couples is recommended.

Women should learn the rhythm of their body and the consistency of cervical mucus at different stages of her cycle. The consistency of cervical mucus is an accurate, easy, and cheap method to determine timing of ovulation. Cervical mucus will change from thick and sticky right after the menstrual period to more clear, slippery, and stretchy at ovulation.

Affirmation

I release blame, shame, guilt, and fear. I am as gentle with myself as I will be with my child.

With long-term zinc supplementation, you have to also supplement with 1–3mg/day of copper to avoid zinc-induced copper deficiency.

INSOMNIA

Symptoms

- Trouble falling/staying asleep
- Waking up too early
- Inability to return to sleep
- Poor sleep quality overall

Root Causes

Depending on the nature of the insomnia and how long it has been present, there are a number of different possible causes to consider.

Adjustment insomnia is short-term and more related to acute psychological stressors or something environmental, like adjusting to sleeping in a new environment. The key for this kind of insomnia is that it should resolve once the stressor(s) is resolved.

The causes for more chronic insomnia fit into to the following categories:

- Psychological (e.g., a period of poor sleep with a growing worry and anxiety about not sleeping well, which contributes to more poor sleep and insomnia.)
- Medications
- Mental health conditions
- Substance abuse and dependence
- Medical conditions (e.g., chronic pain conditions, neurologic diseases, cardiovascular disease)
- Sleep disorders that result in insomnia (e.g., restless leg syndrome, sleep apnea, circadian rhythm disorders)

When the causes listed above don't seem to explain the whole picture, an altered 24-hour cortisol pattern, or decreased cortisol awakening response, may play a role. Hypoglycemia is another reason that people may wake in the night.

Testing

Do a basic screening to rule out other conditions contributing to insomnia.

- CBC
- CMP, Fasting
- TSH
- CRP

Sleep Specific Considerations:

- Nocturnal Hypoxemia Test
- Sleep Study/Polysomnography

Keep a sleep journal for at least two weeks. Record when you go to bed, how many times you woke up, when, why, how long before you went back to sleep, what time you woke up in the morning, and how you felt (refreshed or not).

The cortisol should spike in the morning, at, say, six to eight o'clock, when it's time to wake up, and slowly dissipate over the day. If this pattern is disrupted, tiredness and alertness can come at improper times in the 24-hour period. Consider doing a 24-hour dried urine cortisol that maps the point at each collection to see the cycle as well as the cortisol levels when you wake if this is the case for you.

Treatment

These treatment approaches are things that are generally effective for insomnia. However, it's important to not take something to improve sleep as a symptom without addressing any potential underlying medical conditions. Sleep apnea is a serious condition that needs treatment with a CPAP machine as the underlying causative factors are identified.

Dietary Approach

Some people wake if their blood sugar starts to get low in the night. This can often be remedied by eating a handful of almonds or other protein before bed. You can also leave some almonds by your bed to eat in the middle of the night, which for some people helps them fall back asleep quickly. Eating in a way to improve pre-diabetes or diabetes, if present, will also likely help insomnia. There's more on this in the diabetes section (page 80).

It's a good idea to avoid caffeine and alcohol in the evenings. Both of these can disrupt sleep or worsen an already present problem. Alcohol especially should be avoided with sleep apnea.

Herbs/Supplements

- Magnesium – 300–600mg daily at bedtime
- Vitamin B Complex – one serving daily
- L-theanine – 200–400mg 30 minutes before bed
- Melatonin – 0.3–3mg at bedtime to help falling (not staying) asleep

- Pregnenolone – 10–50mg 30 minutes before bed (If you take this supplement, monitor your sex hormones with your doctor regularly at baseline and for at least the first three to six months.)

INSOMNIA HERBAL TINCTURE FORMULA

Passionflower (*Passiflora incarnata*)
Lemon Balm (*Melissa officinalis*)
Skullcap (*Scutellaria lateriflora*)
Valerian (*Valeriana officinalis*)
Hops (*Humulus lupulus*)
Kava Kava (*Piper methysticum*)

Mix 20% Passionflower, 20% Lemon Balm, 15% Skullcap, 15% Valerian, 15% Hops, 15% Kava Kava. Take 2–5 droppersful at bedtime.

These herbs are all also available individually in capsule form and work well by themselves or in combination. Valerian and Kava Kava are stronger herbs and should be avoided with other sedative medications and alcohol.

Lifestyle Changes

Take healthy measures to improve sleep. Implement a sleep routine and start it around the same time every night. Remove the TV from your room and avoid stimulating activities, including using a mobile device, for an hour before bedtime. A daily practice of meditation or sitting in reflection fits well here, too.

Avoid vigorous exercise right before bed, but otherwise, regular exercise will help improve sleep.

Autogenics training is a technique that you can practice, and over time, can help you change your physiology to improve sleep.

Hypnosis may also be worth a try. Guided hypnosis and self-hypnosis both may improve sleep.

Affirmation

I am present in my body. I let go of the day and its happenings, letting them drift away.

IRRITABLE BOWEL SYNDROME (IBS)

Symptoms

- Generalized abdominal pain
- Constipation and/or diarrhea
- Pain with bowel movements
- Abdominal bloating/distention

The pain of irritable bowel syndrome (IBS) usually varies from time to time, both in character and intensity. It's often not in a specific spot, but more generalized, and can be anything from a dull ache to sharp or burning in character. The lower abdomen and left side are common areas of pain. IBS-related pain can be in conjunction with bowel movements, but it can also be present in isolation. Many people experience decreased pain after bowel movements. Bloating and distention often cause pain as well.

Some people experiencing IBS may only have constipation or diarrhea, whereas others have relatively consistent alternations between the two.

Root Causes

IBS is functional in character. This means that there isn't, at least that we know of, a specific disease pathology or anatomical abnormality. Instead, the function of the intestines and its related parts are altered. There are lots of contributing factors and differing ideas as to the exact cause. These are potential underlying mechanisms and causes for consideration for anyone with IBS.

- Decreased or increased bowel transit (how fast food moves through)
- Altered gut motility
- Hypersensitivity of the bowel muscle and nerves
- Altered gut immune function
- After severe acute intestinal infection
- Chronic gut infection
- Gut dysbiosis
- Small intestinal bacterial overgrowth (SIBO)
- Leaky gut/intestinal permeability
- Food intolerance

Testing

- CBC
- CMP
- TSH
- CRP
- Fecal Calprotectin
- Fecal Lactoferrin
- ANA
- pANCA

- ASCA
- Celiac Disease
- Ova and Parasite x3
- Clostridium Difficile
- Comprehensive Stool Analysis
- Food Elimination/Re-Challenge to assess for intolerances/sensitivities

Other Considerations

- In Depth Stool Pathogen Test (PCR testing for a wide range of organisms)
- SIBO Breath Test
- Colonoscopy
- Ultrasound or other imaging if structural abnormalities are suspected

Treatment

It's always helpful to find something on testing that we can specifically address. Unfortunately, that doesn't always happen, so treatment needs to focus largely on supporting and improving gut and nervous system function.

Dietary Approach

There are different dietary approaches to consider, depending on the individual and how severe the symptoms are. If not already cleaning up the diet as mentioned in chapter 2 with eating whole foods and plant-based, start there.

- Elemental Diet – If really flared up, or also have SIBO, and things won't calm down, using for one to two weeks may help.
- Low-FODMAP Diet – This isn't meant to be a forever diet, but may help calm down periods of intense symptoms and get things to a more manageable place.
- Avoid lactose, fructose, sucrose, and sorbitol.
- Fiber to Tolerance – This approach, in conjunction with adequate water intake, should help symptoms in the long run. Work up slowly to allow the intestines to adapt, as too much bulk may stretch the intestines and cause pain.

- Chew 1–2 tsp of fennel and/or caraway seeds after meals and keep them on hand to chew for relief from pain and discomfort from gas and cramping.

For IBS in particular, a fairly broad food elimination diet can help reveal what's contributing to your symptoms. The premise is to eliminate a large number of foods for at least a couple of weeks. If symptoms improve, you know something you eliminated was contributing or causing the symptoms. You then slowly add one food back in at a time, leaving three days after the addition, to see if symptoms get aggravated. If not, that food is fine and you try the next one. You can eliminate one food, or 30 foods. This experiment obviously gets more difficult with the more foods eliminated. So, I often recommend people start with eliminating soy, dairy, gluten, wheat, potato, egg, and corn, as these are the most common culprits. If symptoms don't improve after two weeks of elimination of these foods, then broaden the elimination to other foods.

Herbs/Supplements

- Broad-Spectrum Probiotic – If this doesn't help, try a soil-based probiotic.
- Magnesium – 150–300mg twice daily
- Digestive Bitters – 5–10 drops on the back of the tongue 5–15 minutes before meals, or three times daily

IBS PAIN HERBAL TINCTURE FORMULA

Fennel (*Foeniculum vulgare*)
Wild Yam (*Dioscorea villosa*)
California Poppy (*Eschscholzia californica*)
Skullcap (*Scutellaria lateriflora*)
Lemon Balm (*Melissa officinalis*)
Cramp Bark (*Viburnum opulus*)

Mix 25% Fennel, 20% Wild Yam, 20% California Poppy, 15% Skullcap, 10% Lemon Balm, 10% Cramp Bark. Take 2–5 droppersful two to three times daily as needed.

IBS HERBAL TINCTURE FORMULA

Milky Oats (*Avena sativa*)
Passionflower (*Passiflora incarnata*)
Turmeric (*Curcuma longa*)
Dandelion Leaf (*Taraxacum officinale*)
Ginger (*Zingiber officinalis*)

Mix 30% Milky Oats, 30% Passionflower, 20% Turmeric, 15% Dandelion Leaf, 5% Ginger. Take 2–4 droppersful two to three times daily for at least six to 12 weeks.

Lifestyle Changes

Poor quality or not enough sleep impairs decision-making and judgment. People with better sleep are able to choose healthier foods and better fight sugar cravings. Sleep also helps us be more resilient on all levels through the cellular restorative processes and nervous system restoration. For these reasons, optimizing sleep can improve IBS.

For many people, symptom flares can be directly correlated to emotional distress. Emotions aren't the problem, but how we process and internalize them can be. Counseling and mindfulness meditations are great body awareness and stress management approaches.

Lastly, heart rate variability training balances the autonomic nervous system, which controls the bowels.

Affirmation

I can digest the events of my daily life with ease and let go of what doesn't serve me just as easily.

LEAKY GUT/INTESTINAL PERMEABILITY

Symptoms

- Fatigue
- Brain fog
- Depression
- Irritable bowel syndrome (IBS)
- Food intolerances, often increasing in number over time

Some conditions that may make one consider leaky gut are autoimmune conditions, developmental disorders such as autism, liver diseases, asthma, eczema, and inflammatory bowel disease.

If you name nearly any symptom, it can be hypothesized how leaky gut could play a role. For this reason, it's always worth consideration.

Root Causes

The intestines are the barrier between our outside and inside worlds, much like our skin. Only certain things are supposed to get through; otherwise inflammation and immune reactions tend to ensue. Permeability can be increased everywhere from the stomach to the colon. Potential causes for leaky gut are alcohol intake, nonsteroidal anti-inflammatory drugs (NSAIDs), aspirin, bacterial gut infections, proton pump inhibitors (PPIs), and chemotherapy drugs. If medications and alcohol intake don't seem to explain things, consider chronic gut infections and food intolerances as the cause. Inflammation from these things can increase gut permeability.

Testing

- Lactulose/Mannitol Test
- Comprehensive Stool Analysis
- Food Elimination/Re-Challenge Diet

Treatment

Remove the offending agents first. You can't repair the gut barrier if the triggering substance or organism isn't addressed.

Dietary Approach

- Eliminate sugar.
- Eliminate food intolerances.
- Eat foods high in soluble fiber daily.
- Incorporate ginger and turmeric into more foods for anti-inflammatory benefits.
- Increase bioflavonoid content in the diet.

Herbs/Supplements

- Vitamin C – 1g two to three times daily
- Zinc* – 15mg daily
- Broad Spectrum Probiotic daily
- L-Glutamine – 3g two to three times daily
- Curcumin – 1–2g daily
- Digestive Bitters – 5–10 drops on the back of the tongue, three times daily, ideally 5–15 minutes before meals
- DGL, marshmallow root powder, and aloe mixture. Many specialty products contain these. If mixing yourself, do equal parts, with 1 tbsp per 8–12oz water. Drink twice daily.

Lifestyle Changes

Maintain regular bowel movements. Doing so will mean increasing fiber to 30–50g daily and getting adequate water intake. Address constipation if present. Data suggests simply keeping regular bowel movements may decrease intestinal permeability. A good goal is two to three well-formed and easy to pass stools.

Affirmation

I have healthy boundaries in my relationships and with the outside world.

MENOPAUSE

Symptoms

- Increasingly irregular and infrequent periods
- Hot flashes/night sweats
- Breast tenderness
- Mood changes
- Poor concentration
- Memory difficulties
- Depression and/or anxiety
- Vaginal tissue atrophy
- Vaginal dryness
- More frequent urinary tract infections

Menopause is the transition to the absence of a menstrual cycle. As the transition progresses, there are months between cycles until the last cycle happens. Menopausal symptoms can vary from six months to 10 years. Some women will experience little to no symptoms aside from cycle changes.

Root Causes

Menopause is the normal transition a woman goes through, usually starting in her late 40s to early 50s, and it typically progresses over a period of years. During this transition, the ovaries stop producing the sex hormones estrogen and progesterone. Most of the symptoms happen during the transitional years when the hormones are fluctuating.

Testing

Testing usually isn't needed for diagnosis. The following tests will help rule out imbalances not necessarily due to perimenopause or pregnancy.

- Fractionated Estrogens
- Progesterone
- Sex Hormone Binding Globulin (SHBG)
- CMP – primarily for liver function tests
- Human Chorionic Gonadotropin (hCG) (pregnancy test)

Other Considerations

Follicle-stimulating hormone (FSH)—Once elevated consistently, and a year has passed since the last menstrual period, this is diagnostic of menopause.

Treatment

Treatment is focused on hormonal balancing and hormone detoxification.

Dietary Approach

- Avoid caffeine, including tea, and chocolate. Doing so is shown to improve symptoms in the majority of women.
- Get 30–50g fiber daily.
- Decrease or eliminate alcohol altogether.
- Increase Brassica family plants.
- Avoid BPA. Discard all plastic water bottles and food storage.

Herbs/Supplements

- N-Acetylcysteine – 600mg one to two times daily
- Selenium – 100mcg daily

Drink tea of these phytoestrogen plants often, either individually or in combination. Steep 1 tbsp of herb per cup of hot water for about 5 minutes. Licorice root needs to be decocted instead of steeped.

Red Clover (*Trifolium pratense*)
Calendula (*Calendula officinalis*)
Plantain (*Plantago spp.*)
Licorice (*Glycyrrhiza glabra*)

MENOPAUSE HERBAL TINCTURE FORMULA

Chaste Tree (*Vitex agnus castus*)
Dong Quai (*Angelica sinensis*)
Dandelion Root (*Taraxacum officinalis*)
Burdock (*Arctium lappa*)
Motherwort (*Leonurus cardiaca*)
Black Cohosh (*Actaea racemosa*)

Mix 20% Chaste Tree, 20% Dong Quai, 15% Dandelion Root, 15% Burdock, 15% Motherwort, 15% Black Cohosh. Take 2–4 droppersful two to three times daily.

Lifestyle Changes

Maintaining regular exercise is important. This is a time also to start weight-bearing exercise. Bone density will decrease as estrogen levels drop, and this form of exercise is one way to maintain bone density. Regular exercise also helps the body detoxify hormones and improves hormonal regulation.

The menopausal transition is not so much about hormones, but a life transition to the elder and the matriarch. Depending on how you've defined yourself up until now, this transition may be difficult to accept. Trust in this natural process, and get the support you need along the way.

Affirmation

My feminine nature is maturing. I am claiming my rightful place as the archetypal wise woman.

MULTIPLE SCLEROSIS

Symptoms

The most common early symptoms are:

- Paresthesia, which can involve one or more extremities, the trunk, or one side of the face
- Weakness/difficulty with function of a leg/hand
- Visual disturbances (e.g., partial loss of vision and pain in one eye, double vision, or scotomas)

Other common symptoms include:

- Bladder control problems
- Fatigue
- Heat intolerance
- Muscle weakness/easy muscle fatigue
- Numbness/tingling
- Pain
- Vertigo
- Disturbances of gait

Many other neurologic symptoms are possible, depending on what part of the brain or spinal cord is affected.

There are four different patterns of symptom presentation in multiple sclerosis (MS):

- Relapsing-Remitting is where symptoms come and go at varying intervals, often with months or even years between relapses.
- Primary Progressive is where there is a steady and progressive worsening of symptoms with no remission.
- Secondary Progressive is where there is relapsing and remission initially, later followed by steady progression.
- Progressive Relapsing is where the disease is progressive and then there are unexpected remissions and relapses.

Root Causes

MS is an inflammatory disorder mediated by the immune system. This inflammation attacks the myelin in areas of the brain and sometimes the spinal cord. Myelin shows up as plaques on an MRI and is used for nerve conduction. The various symptoms occur in those areas of the nervous system with decreased conduction.

Various causes are possible, and nothing concrete is known at this time. MS is likely the result of multiple factors playing in concert. Primary considerations for contribution to illness from a naturopathic perspective should be:

- Viral infection (e.g., Epstein-Barr)
- Gut dysbiosis and pathogens
- Leaky gut/intestinal permeability
- Heavy metal toxicity (e.g., aluminum, mercury)
- Other toxin burden (e.g., pesticides, industrial chemicals)
- History of inflammatory behaviors (e.g., smoking, heavy alcohol use, inflammatory diet)
- Chronic infections
- Leaky blood brain barrier (causes neuro-inflammation)

Testing

A comprehensive neurologic evaluation by a specialist and MRI are important for the diagnosis. Other tests to look for different contributing factors include:

- CBC
- CMP
- Methylmalonic Acid
- CRP
- ESR
- Neutrophil/Lymphocyte Ratio (NLR)
- Fasting Lipid Panel
- Vitamin D
- ANA with reflex cascade

Other Considerations

- Urine Toxic Metals
- Comprehensive Stool Analysis
- Comprehensive Nutrient Panel
- Genetic SNP Panel
- Pathogens like reactivated Epstein-Barr Virus, Cytomegalovirus Virus, Lyme Disease, and other tickborne diseases, if other tests aren't showing much.

Treatment

Dietary Approach

The first steps should be integrating a sustainable, anti-inflammatory diet into your life. Once this diet is a state of normalcy, it is worth considering a ketogenic diet for a couple months to a year to see what changes in symptoms and imaging take place. Before making this change, educate yourself on a ketogenic diet. I also recommend working with a professional who is knowledgeable in this area.

Intermittent fasting is an approach you can take now, in addition to a whole-food, plant-based diet to balance blood sugar and improve cellular function.

Herbs/Supplements

- Vitamin B Complex – one serving daily
- Magnesium – 150–300mg twice daily
- N-Acetylcysteine – 600mg one to two times daily
- Selenium – 100mcg daily
- Fish Oil – 1–2g daily
- Curcumin – 2–4g daily
- *Bacopa monnieri* – 500mg one to two times daily
- Pregnenolone – 10–50mg daily at bedtime
- Broad Spectrum Probiotic – daily

BRAIN BLOOD FLOW HERBAL TINCTURE FORMULA

Gotu Kola (*Centella asiatica*)
Rosemary (*Rosmarinus officinalis*)
Ginkgo (*Ginkgo biloba*)
Ginger (*Zingiber officinalis*)

Mix 35% Gotu Kola, 30% Rosemary, 30% Ginkgo, 5% Ginger. Take 2–4 droppersful three times daily.

IMMUNE MODULATING HERBAL TINCTURE FORMULA

Siberian Ginseng *(Eleutherococcus senticosus)*
Astragalus *(Astragalus membranaceus)*
Devil's Club *(Oplopanax horridus)*
Ashwagandha *(Withania somnifera)*
Licorice *(Glycyrrhiza glabra)*

Mix 25% Siberian Ginseng, 25% Astragalus, 20% Devil's Club, 20% Ashwagandha, 10% Licorice. Take 2–4 droppersful two to three times daily long term. I recommend taking this as long as it supports remission.

Lifestyle Changes

A healthy lifestyle on all fronts is vital when living with MS. Just focusing on diet or supplements, for example, likely won't achieve your desired results. Exercise, eliminating inflammatory behaviors, daily meditation, and stress reduction and management are all part of the holistic approach.

Start optimizing and prioritizing sleep. The better your sleep is, the better your nervous system will function.

Refrain from smoking and excessive alcohol consumption. Eliminating alcohol entirely is the best route to take.

Neurofeedback is likely to help with various symptoms of MS, like depression, cognitive function, and fatigue.

Take a team approach for treatment. A neurologist, naturopathic doctor, physical therapist, and counselor—in addition to your primary care provider—are all recommended to utilize.

Affirmation

I can regenerate and redefine myself at any time. I embody my authentic self with ease.

OBSESSIVE COMPULSIVE DISORDER (OCD)

Symptoms

Per Medscape.com, obsessions commonly manifest as:

- Contamination
- Safety
- Doubting one's memory or perception
- Scrupulosity (need to do the right thing; fear of committing a transgression, often religious)
- Need for order or symmetry
- Unwanted, intrusive sexual/aggressive thoughts

The website lists common compulsions as:

- Cleaning/washing
- Checking (e.g., locks, stove, iron, safety of children)
- Counting/repeating actions a certain number of times or until it "feels right"
- Arranging objects
- Touching/tapping objects
- Hoarding
- Confessing/seeking reassurance
- List making

The compulsions are usually a behavior that eases the anxiety around the obsession.

There are also commonly other disorders present with OCD, such as eating disorders, tic disorders, and ADHD. There can also be skin lesions present from obsessive picking and scratching.

Root Causes

Neurotransmitters and the brain's response to them appear to play a large role in OCD. Serotonin and dopamine abnormalities in particular seem to be involved. There are also thought to be abnormalities in the part of the brain that is excitatory in nature, the glutamate system. Other considerations are group A strep infection, which afterward may lead to these symptoms in children. This is termed Post Autoimmune Neuropsychiatric Disorders Associated with Streptococcal Infections (PANDAS), and possibly in more rare cases, head injury or stimulant abuse may be causative.

Testing

Get evaluated by a specialist, such as a psychologist or a psychiatrist, to get an appropriate diagnosis. The Yale-Brown Obsessive-Compulsive Scale (Y-BOCS) is an easily accessible questionnaire used to rate the severity of OCD in adolescents.

If ADHD (page 58) or other conditions are present, look at those specific sections for testing and treatment approaches.

Treatment

Conventional treatment is focused on therapy and medications, which includes selective serotonin reuptake inhibitors (SSRIs). With a holistic and natural approach, we can increase serotonin, calm the nervous system and anxiety (common with OCD), and decrease the glutamate (excitatory) activity of the central nervous system. This is a well-rounded approach that makes more sense than simply focusing on one or two areas.

Dietary Approach

- Avoid caffeine, including tea, and chocolate.
- Avoid monosodium glutamate (MSG).
- Ensure adequate protein, at least 1–1.2g/kg body weight daily.

Herbs/Supplements

- N-Acetylcysteine – 600mg two to three times daily
- Vitamin B Complex – one serving daily
- Magnesium – 150–300mg one to two times daily
- Taurine – 500mg two to three times daily

OCD HERBAL TINCTURE FORMULA

St. John's Wort *(Hypericum perforatum)* *
Passionflower *(Passiflora incarnata)*
California Poppy *(Eschscholzia californica)*
Milky Oats *(Avena sativa)*
Skullcap *(Scutellaria lateriflora)*

Mix 50% St. John's Wort, 20% Passionflower, 10% California Poppy, 10% Milky Oats, 10% Skullcap. Take 2–4 droppersful three times daily.

Lifestyle Changes

A healthy sleep routine is vital in helping the brain function as optimally as possible; getting seven to eight hours a night is recommended. Avoid things that effect sleep quality, such as alcohol, excessive "screen time," and stimulants.

Neurofeedback has been shown in small trials to be effective for OCD. A combination of the natural therapeutics listed here, coupled with neurofeedback, is recommended.

Exposure and response prevention (ERP), a type of cognitive behavioral therapy (CBT), is an evidence-based approach to essentially desensitize oneself to the mental effects of the obsession.

Affirmation

I feel my feet on the ground and connect to the earth. I am cared for. I am safe.

---

* *St. John's Wort interacts with certain medications like SSRI's. Check for interactions if taking other medications and work with a trained practitioner.*

OSTEOPENIA & OSTEOPOROSIS

Symptoms

- No symptoms unless a fracture occurs, in which case pain from the fracture is expected
- Increased risk for fragility fractures (happens after less force than would normally be expected to break a bone)

  Common areas for fragility fractures are the wrist, hip, pelvis, and spine.

Root Causes

Osteopenia and osteoporosis are two different severities of the same condition. Osteopenia means decreased bone mass, and as such, the bone also gets weaker. Osteoporosis is the same thing, but with more severe bone loss and weakness.

Bone is always being built and broken down. We build the most bone density in our adolescent and young adult years, with an average peak bone density around age 30. After this point, we all have a steady decline in bone mass.

Undernutrition, or malnutrition, at a young age is a major predisposing factor. Anorexia as a teenager and young adult is one of the worst-case scenarios for later developing osteoporosis, because this is the time when bone is supposed to be building.

Nutrient deficiencies, such as calcium, magnesium, phosphorus, and vitamin D, can predispose to osteoporosis. Bone mass is also greatly influenced by the presence or lack of estrogen. Bone breaks down more without estrogen present, hence, there is a greater bone loss in women after menopause.

Other risk factors for osteoporosis include:

- Immobilization
- Low body mass index
- Wide variety of genetic conditions
- Tobacco and alcohol use
- Family history
- Corticosteroids and many other medications
- Chronic illnesses of many types

Finally, many heavy metals such as lead, tin, aluminum, and cadmium can replace other minerals in bone and result in a weak structure.

Testing

Dual-energy x-ray absorptiometry (DXA) is a special x-ray that is used to measure bone density. The readings come back as low positive, or negative numbers. The lower the number, the lower the density. Results are given as T scores. A T score of < −1 but > −2.5 is a diagnosis of osteopenia. A T score of <−2.5 is osteoporosis.

- CBC
- CMP
- TSH
- Vitamin D
- Serum Calcium
- Serum Magnesium
- RBC Magnesium
- Serum Phosphorus
- Parathyroid Hormone
- Testosterone in men
- Estrogen in women
- 24-hour urine calcium and creatinine

If there is a problem with unexplained weight loss and/or malabsorption, rule out celiac disease (page 68) and Crohn's disease (page 72), and read those sections, respectively.

Treatment

Dietary Approach

- Avoid excessive caffeine.
- Eliminate refined sugar.
- Consume an anti-inflammatory diet.
- Avoid processed and fast foods.
- Decrease or eliminate alcohol altogether.
- Avoid BPA. Discard all plastic water bottles and food storage.
- Eat a couple of servings of dark, leafy vegetables daily.
- Eat 7–10 servings of vegetables daily.

Herbs/Supplements

A variety of minerals play a role in bone health. I recommend taking a multimineral that contains copper (1–3mg), manganese (5–15mg), zinc (15mg), silicon (1–5mg), and strontium (2–5mg). The following minerals may be present in the multimineral, but the total daily intake should equal what is listed in this section, so you may have to take more than what's present in the multimineral supplement.

There are also many osteoporosis supplements that contain all of these minerals in adequate amounts.

- Vitamin D3 – 2000–5000IU daily
- Calcium citrate – 500mg two times daily
- Magnesium – 300–600mg daily
- Vitamin K2 – 45mcg daily, or Vitamin K1 – 500–1000mcg daily
- Vitamin C – 1g one to three times daily
- Vitamin B Complex – one serving daily

Lifestyle Changes

Incorporate safe weight-bearing and non-weight-bearing exercise into your weekly routine. See a physical therapist (PT) to improve balance. If you prevent falls, you prevent fractures. Yoga is another activity that improves balance. Tai chi improves balance and decrease falls as well.

Affirmation

I am strong and adaptable, like a grown fir tree. I bend with life, always returning to my center.

PARKINSON'S DISEASE

Symptoms

The most common first sign of Parkinson's disease (PD) is a resting tremor in an upper extremity. Other symptoms include:

- Softening of the voice
- Decreased sense of smell
- General weakness
- Decreased facial expression
- Sleep disturbances
- Depression
- Slow cognition
- Constipation
- Sweating

As PD progresses, movements become slower and the gait (walking) becomes shorter and more difficult. Muscle functions also begin to become more rigid, there is difficulty in dexterity with the hands, and posture tends to be more bent over.

Root Causes

Genetics account for about 10 percent of PD cases. The other 90 percent are presumably from a combination of environmental factors and genetic susceptibility. What results in PD, regardless of the underlying causes, is a drastic decrease in the cells of the brain that produce dopamine. The symptoms are all secondary to this loss.

Various chemical toxicities are clearly associated with the development of PD, and oxidative stressors are hypothesized to be a major player. Examples of oxidative stressors can be diabetes or from a decrease in body antioxidant levels, in particular glutathione. Pesticides, herbicides, and various solvent chemicals are highly associated with PD formation as well. Iron is a heavy metal that can contribute to PD when present in excess.

Testing

Appropriate neurologic testing from a neurologist is an important first step if PD is suspected. Other tests to assess baseline health:

- CBC
- CMP
- TSH
- Ferritin
- Vitamin D
- hsCRP
- Neutrophil/Lymphocyte Ratio (NLR)
- Heavy Metals Urine Testing

Treatment

PD is a perfect example of why we need to eat a whole-food, clean, plant-based diet for overall health. Doing so provides adequate antioxidants and decreases toxin exposure. Along with approaches that promote normal body detoxification pathways, this diet is the foundation to prevent and slow PD disease progression.

Dietary Approach

- Eliminate refined sugar.
- Eat organic, at least the Dirty Dozen by the EWG as well as wheat.
- Eat 7–10 servings of vegetables daily.
- Get 30–50g fiber daily.
- Decrease or eliminate alcohol altogether.
- Get adequate protein daily, at least 1–1.2g/kg body weight daily.
- Eat protein with each meal, especially in the morning.

Herbs/Supplements

- Vitamin D3 – 2000–5000IU daily
- Vitamin C – 1g two to three times daily
- Vitamin E – 250mg daily
- Vitamin B Complex – one serving daily
- Magnesium – 300mg daily
- N-Acetylcysteine – 600mg two to three times daily
- Selenium – 100mcg daily
- CoQ10 – 1000–1500mg daily
- Broad Spectrum Probiotic – daily

Sublingual and intravenous glutathione are other options that may prove beneficial, especially in early PD. Discuss these options with your neurologist as well as a naturopathic doctor to decide what's best for you.

Lifestyle Changes

Practice good sleep hygiene. As sleep disturbance is often part of PD, and addressing this issue will likely help improve daily function on cognitive and physical levels.

Fall prevention is another important consideration, as PD progressively affects gait and balance. Use good lighting, eliminate texture or level changes in floors, and keep walking areas as free of obstacles as possible.

Tai chi has been shown to increase balance and decrease falls.

For detoxification, sweat for 20 minutes, at least three times a week and indefinitely. If sauna access isn't possible, hot baths work as well.

Affirmation

I openly experience my emotions, and I am fully present in my life.

POLYCYSTIC OVARY SYNDROME (PCOS)

Symptoms

- Irregular/absent menstrual cycle
- Weight gain/difficulty losing weight
- Excess hair growth (i.e., upper lip, chin, back, etc.)
- Insulin resistance and high insulin production
- Sleep disturbance
- Obstructive sleep apnea
- Infertility (PCOS is one of the top causes in the United States)
- Early development of puberty signs in children
- Fatigue
- Cysts in the ovaries (these cysts can also be absent)

Root Causes

Women with PCOS have abnormalities in how their body metabolizes estrogen and testosterone as well as in the production of testosterone. It is typical for there to be increased insulin production, and also a resistance to insulin, which leads to metabolic syndrome or diabetes. The weight gain associated with PCOS causes this insulin resistance to be worse and can further alter the hormonal functions. Many genes have been researched and associated with PCOS. There is also a strong heritability noted with PCOS.

This condition, at this time, appears to be largely genetic in origin, but there are a great deal of environmental factors that can play into the severity of the condition. Quality of diet and exercise levels have a significant role to play in symptom severity. Also, many environmental toxins affect hormone metabolism and insulin resistance.

Testing

- Fractionated Estrogens
- Progesterone
- Testosterone, free and total
- Dihydrotestosterone (DHT)
- Prolactin
- SHBG
- DHEA-S
- Follicle-Stimulating Hormone (FSH)
- Luteinizing Hormone (LH)
- CMP, Fasting
- CBC

- Fasting Lipid Panel
- Hemoglobin A1C
- Insulin
- hsCRP
- TSH
- hCG to rule out pregnancy

It is recommended hormone labs be drawn between day five to nine of the menstrual cycle (if cycling), in the early morning.

Other Considerations

A comprehensive hormone panel with urinary metabolites is the best way to get a deeper understanding of hormonal imbalances and how to treat them.

Treatment

Treatment is focused on hormonal balancing, hormone detoxification, and blood sugar management.

Dietary Approach

- Eat a diet that supports balanced blood sugar and healthy insulin sensitivity. Follow the dietary information given in the diabetes section (page 80).
- Avoid processed and fast foods.
- Avoid BPA. Discard all plastic water bottles and food storage.
- Intermittent fasting can help with blood sugar management.
- Eating soy a couple of times a week may help due to the phytoestrogen effects.

Herbs/Supplements

- Chromium – 200–1000mcg daily
- Multivitamin – one daily
- Vitamin D3 – 2000–5000IU daily
- N-Acetylcysteine – 600mg one to two times daily
- Selenium – 100mcg daily
- Berberine – 500mg two to three times daily depending on level of blood sugar imbalance
- Magnesium – 300mg one to two times daily

Drink tea of these phytoestrogen plants often, either individually or in combination. Steep 1 tbsp of herb per cup of hot water for about 5 minutes. Licorice root needs to be decocted instead of steeped.

Red Clover (*Trifolium pratense*)
Calendula (*Calendula officinalis*)
Plantain (*Plantago spp.*)
Licorice (*Glycyrrhiza glabra*)

PCOS HERBAL TINCTURE FORMULA

Chaste Tree (*Vitex agnus-castus*)
Dandelion Root (*Taraxacum officinale*)
Schisandra (*Schisandra chinensis*)
Burdock (*Arctium lappa*)
Milk Thistle (*Silybum marianum*)

Mix 40% Chaste Tree, 20% Dandelion Root, 20% Schisandra, 10% Burdock, 10% Milk Thistle. 2–3 droppersful two to three times daily.

The herbal support for diabetes will be beneficial as well.

Lifestyle Changes

Aside from diet, exercise is the area to put energy into the most. Exercise will help blood sugar control and hormone balance and detoxification as well as weight loss. With PCOS, you have to work harder than many others to keep your metabolism functioning in a healthy way.

Getting enough sleep (seven to eight hours a night) will help in making choices congruent with your goals. Research has shown that neglecting sleep leads to giving in to sugar cravings. In essence, not getting enough sleep decreases our mental and emotional resilience.

Affirmation

I feel balanced and beautiful in my body. I accept myself with love.

PREMENSTRUAL SYNDROME (PMS)

Symptoms

- Mood swings/irritability
- Depression and/or anxiety
- Breast tenderness
- Swelling of extremities
- Food cravings
- Headaches
- Memory problems
- Hot flashes
- Bowel habit changes
- Nausea
- Sleep problems

PMS symptoms can vary from mild discomfort to severe enough to significantly affect one's life and well-being. Symptoms arise in the days before, and in worse cases, more than a week before the menstrual period begins. Symptoms either improve with the start of the period or can carry on until the finish.

Root Causes

The exact mechanisms of what causes PMS aren't known. PMS occurs in the luteal phase, the second half of the menstrual cycle, after ovulation. This is the phase when estrogen is dropping and progesterone is rising at first, then dropping before the period begins.

Smoking and obesity are both two well-known risk factors. Women with a body mass index (BMI) greater than 30 are three times more likely to have PMS. Smokers are two times as likely.

There is a hypothesis that low serotonin may play a role, because PMS often responds to treatments that increase serotonin. Magnesium and calcium deficiency are other potential contributors.

Testing

- CBC
- CMP
- RBC Magnesium
- TSH
- Ferritin
- hsCRP

Other Considerations

Hormone cycle mapping may be helpful if PMS is not changing with the following recommended treatments, or if there are also other cycle abnormalities present. Testing estrogen and progesterone specifically in the late luteal phase may also be useful.

Treatment

PMS can not only improve but also resolve. Put energy into the foundations of health, namely diet and exercise, as well as the other recommendations here. Within a few months, there should be noticeable positive change.

Dietary Approach

- Eliminate refined sugar.
- Avoid BPA. Discard all plastic water bottles and food storage.
- Decrease or eliminate alcohol.
- Eliminate food intolerances.
- Increase Brassica family plants in the diet substantially.
- Get 30–50g fiber daily.
- Eat 7–10 servings of vegetables daily.

Herbs/Supplements

- Vitamin B Complex – one serving daily
- Magnesium – 150–300mg twice daily
- N-Acetylcysteine – 600mg two to three times daily
- Selenium – 100mcg daily

PMS HERBAL TINCTURE FORMULA

Chaste Tree *(Vitex agnus-castus)*
Dong Quai *(Angelica sinensis)*
Schisandra *(Schisandra chinensis)*
Dandelion Root *(Taraxacum officinale)*
Burdock *(Arctium lappa)*
Milk Thistle *(Silybum marianum)*

Mix 25% Chaste Tree, 25% Dong Quai, 15% Schisandra, 15% Dandelion Root, 10% Burdock, 10% Milk Thistle. Take 2–4 droppersful two to three times daily.

If this formula doesn't seem to help, or if things worsen, try taking a Chaste Tree standardized extract, around 200mg daily.

Lifestyle Changes

As mentioned in the cause section, smoking and obesity play large roles in predisposing to PMS. Make efforts to quit smoking. Develop lifestyle habits that will support a healthy weight, which are largely movement, sleep, diet, and stress management.

Affirmation

I move with the cycles of the earth and the moon, without resistance or fear to what transition brings.

RESTLESS LEG SYNDROME (RLS)

Symptoms

- Irresistible urge to move the legs or arms (or less commonly, other body parts)
- Paresthesia (e.g., creeping or crawling sensations)
- Pain in the upper or lower extremities

RLS symptoms tend to be worse at rest, toward bedtime, and in bed. These symptoms often interrupt the quantity and quality of sleep.

Root Causes

RLS can be secondary to many other conditions. Nutrient deficiencies, neurologic conditions like Parkinson's disease or multiple sclerosis, kidney disease, diabetes, and liver disease are all possible primary causes.

RLS can be present without other factors and the cause isn't known, but it is thought to possibly be due to abnormalities in dopamine transmission in the brain.

Other scenarios that may result in RLS are stimulant abuse, various drug withdrawals, and pregnancy.

Testing

Testing is for general health screening and checking certain nutrient status.

- CBC
- CMP
- Lipid Panel
- hsCRP
- TSH
- Iron Panel with Ferritin
- RBC Magnesium
- Hemoglobin A1C

Treatment

We want to tonify/strengthen the calming side of the nervous system, and also provide nutrients that support muscle and nervous system relaxation.

Dietary Approach

- Eat 7–10 servings of vegetables daily.
- Increase legumes and other high magnesium foods.

Study the diabetes section (page 80) for advice if blood sugar control is a problem. Improving blood sugar will help RLS.

Herbs/Supplements

- Vitamin E – 250mg daily
- Vitamin B Complex – one serving daily
- Magnesium – 300–600mg daily at bedtime, or split into two daily doses
- Glycine – 500–1000mg at bedtime
- GABA – 500mg at bedtime
- Taurine – 500mg once or twice daily

These are mild, calming, generally very safe, herbs to experiment with:

Skullcap *(Scutellaria lateriflora)*
Passionflower *(Passiflora incarnata)*
California Poppy *(Eschscholzia californica)*
Lemon Balm *(Melissa officinalis)*
Chamomile *(Matricaria recutita)*
Catnip *(Nepeta cataria)*
Vervain *(Verbena officinalis)*
Lavender *(Lavandula angustifolia)*

Stronger herbs that help with sleep and may help RLS at night, if the above herbal recommendations aren't working:

Valerian *(Valeriana officinalis)*
Kava Kava *(Piper methysticum)*

These herbs may increase the effects of other sedative medications. Use appropriate caution and seek the advice of a trained professional here.

Lifestyle Changes

Exercise may help RLS a great deal. Start working out to where your muscles burn and begin to feel tired. High-intensity interval training (HIIT), walking/running stairs, or leg presses are all options. If there are nutrient deficiencies, this kind of exercise could exacerbate RLS, but with appropriate diet and nutrient supplementation, it should not be a problem.

Epsom salt baths and topically applied magnesium gel may also help.

Affirmation

I express my truth with confidence.

RHEUMATOID ARTHRITIS (RA)

Symptoms

- Joint pain, stiffness, and/or swelling

Any joint can be affected by RA, but the most common ones are the ankles, knees, hips, the wrist, elbow, and shoulder, and the proximal (closer to the wrist/ankle) finger, hand and feet joints. Other symptoms can include:

- Fatigue/weakness
- Low grade fever
- Decreased appetite

As the disease progresses untreated, joint deformities ensue. Organs such as the skin, heart, and lungs can also be affected by RA.

Root Causes

RA is an autoimmune (AI) condition. The body produces antibodies that create inflammation and joint destruction. As the joints deteriorate, obvious deformities and decreased joint function take place.

AI illness is inflammatory in nature and is often associated with traumatic emotional and physical events, viral or other infections, leaky gut, gut dysbiosis, and in the case of RA, it clearly responds to hormonal differences, such as increasing and decreasing estrogen. Another causative area for consideration is periodontal disease.

Testing

- CBC
- CMP
- CRP
- ESR
- ANA with reflex cascade
- Rheumatoid Factor (RF)

- Anti-Cyclic Citrullinated Peptide (anti-CCP)
- Anti-Mutated Citrullinated Vimentin (anti-MCV)
- X-ray of affected joints

Other Considerations

- Food Elimination/Re-Challenge to assess for intolerances/sensitivities
- Hormone Panel if there are other signs of hormonal imbalance present
- Comprehensive Stool Analysis

Treatment

Dietary Approach

An anti-inflammatory diet is the foundational dietary approach in AI conditions. Eating a variety of legumes, nuts, vegetables, and fruits daily will provide antioxidant compounds that will be protective against tissue damage.

- Identify and eliminate food intolerances.
- Eliminate sugar.
- Eliminate processed and fast foods completely.
- Intermittent fasting for six to 12 weeks to assess for symptom improvement.
- Eat 7–10 servings of vegetables daily.
- Avoid industrial processed seed oils (e.g., cottonseed, soy, corn, etc.).

Herbs/Supplements

- Curcumin – 2g twice daily for acute flares. 1g one to two times daily for maintenance.
- High EPA/DHA Fish Oil – 1–2g daily
- Broad Spectrum Probiotic – daily
- Vitamin B Complex – one serving daily
- Vitamin C – 1g two to three times daily
- Vitamin E – 250mg daily
- Selenium – 100mcg daily
- N-Acetyl Cysteine – 600mg two to three times daily
- Zinc* – 15mg twice daily

*Discontinue supplements after three months, or if rapid improvements happen before that. This is not meant to be used a long term supplement, but to replete potential deficiency.

IMMUNE MODULATING HERBAL TINCTURE FORMULA

Astragalus (*Astragalus membranaceus*)
Siberian Ginseng (*Eleutherococcus senticosus*)
Devil's Club (*Oplopanax horridus*)
Ashwagandha (*Withania somnifera*)
Licorice (*Glycyrrhiza glabra*)

Mix 25% Astragalus, 25% Siberian Ginseng, 20% Devil's Club, 20% Ashwagandha, 10% Licorice. Take 2–4 droppersful two to three times daily long term.

Lifestyle Changes

Even though stiffness and pain typically get in the way, movement is important as it helps preserve range of motion and potentially decrease stiffness. Moving the affected joints while simultaneously utilizing contrast hydrotherapy is highly recommended.

Affirmation

I treat myself with love and respect. I am gentle with myself as I move through the world.

ROSACEA

Symptoms

- Flushing of the face and/or scalp
- Telangiectasia of face
- Papules or pustules
- Coarsening of the skin

The sun, hot weather, hot drinks, alcohol, and strong stressors or emotions can trigger this flushing and redness. There are also ocular (eye) forms of rosacea, which result in inflammation of different parts of the eye.

The rash most commonly involves the cheeks and nose, and importantly for diagnosis, typically covers the space between the nostrils and cheeks, whereas the butterfly rash associated with lupus characteristically does not.

Root Causes

Rosacea is an inflammatory condition. Beyond that, the cause is unknown. Some hypotheses of causation are vascular and blood flow abnormalities, degeneration of the skin protective matrix, chemicals found in different foods and beverages, microbes, increased expression of the iron storage protein ferritin, reactive oxygen species, and others. An association between decreased stomach acid production and rosacea has been observed in studies as far back as 1920.

Testing

- CBC
- CMP, Fasting
- Hemoglobin A1C
- hsCRP
- Ferritin
- ANA with reflex cascade if autoimmune disease is suspected
- Food Elimination/Re-challenge to asses for food intolerances/sensitivities

Other Considerations
Skin biopsy is useful to rule out other conditions.

Treatment

Dietary Approach

The primary recommendation here is to explore potential food intolerances and eliminate them. This is accomplished by eliminating a range of foods for at least two weeks. If symptoms improve with elimination, you know something you removed was contributing. You then add the foods back in one by one, waiting three days between each introduction, seeing if there is an aggravation. Any food can be a culprit, but soy, dairy, potato, corn, wheat, gluten, and egg are the most common. I recommend starting with eliminating those foods.

Herbs/Supplements

- Vitamin C – 1g two to three times daily
- Vitamin D – 2000–5000IU daily
- N-Acetylcysteine – 600mg one to two times daily
- Selenium – 100mcg daily
- Zinc* – 15mg daily
- Digestive bitters – 5–10 drops on the back of the tongue three time daily, ideally 5–15 minutes before meals.

ROSACEA HERBAL TINCTURE FORMULA

Dandelion Root (*Taraxacum officinale*)
Milk Thistle (*Silybum marianum*)
Turmeric (*Curcuma longa*)
Burdock (*Arctium lappa*)
Licorice (*Glycyrrhiza glabra*)

Mix 30% Dandelion Root, 25% Milk Thistle, 25% Turmeric, 15% Burdock, 5% Licorice. Take 1–3 droppersful two to three times daily.

With long-term zinc supplementation, you have to also supplement with 1–3mg/day of copper to avoid zinc-induced copper deficiency.

Lifestyle Changes

Exercising to the point of sweating and getting the heart rate up until you are out of breath will move blood through the organs and skin. Doing so will also start to increase your natural antioxidant systems. Keep regular vigorous exercise in your routine at least two to three times a week.

Affirmation

I am grounded and connected to the earth.

ULCERATIVE COLITIS

Symptoms

- Bloody stools
- Diarrhea
- Lower abdominal pain
- Cramping

Symptoms of ulcerative colitis (UC) are usually remitting and then relapsing in nature. Stools can be well-formed, yet there is usually mucus and/or blood present. Fever is also possible during a UC flare.

Although the colon is the part of the digestive tract affected, there are also other parts of the body outside of the digestive tract that can be affected.

Some of the other complications and disease associations listed by Medscape.com are:

- Uveitis
- Pyoderma gangrenosum
- Pleuritis
- Erythema nodosum
- Ankylosing spondylitis
- Spondyloarthropathies
- Primary sclerosing cholangitis
- Multiple sclerosis
- Immunobullous disease of the skin

Root Causes

UC is an inflammatory bowel disease (IBD). Whereas the other major IBD, Crohn's disease, can affect any part of the digestive tract, UC typically only affects the colon, starting at the rectum and proceeding farther up as time goes on.

UC is autoimmune (AI) in nature. As such, the same general rules apply here, as to the other AI conditions discussed in this book (i.e., Crohn's disease, Hashimoto's thyroiditis, rheumatoid arthritis, etc.). A combination of genetic and environmental factors plays a role. The inflammation in UC causes ulcers in the mucosa of the colon, and this inflammatory damage results in the characteristic bleeding, pain, and loose stools.

Gut infections, dysbiosis, and poor antioxidant status may all play a role in UC as well.

Testing

- CBC
- CMP
- Lipid Panel
- CRP
- ESR
- Fecal Leukocytes
- Fecal Calprotectin
- Fecal Lactoferrin
- pANCA

- ASCA
- Iron Panel with Ferritin
- RBC Magnesium
- Zinc
- Vitamin D
- Food Elimination/Re-Challenge to asses for food intolerances/sensitivities

Other Considerations

Colonoscopy with a biopsy is the best test to confirm diagnosis.

Abdominal x-ray with barium swallow, abdominal CT, and abdominal MRI can all be useful depending on disease severity.

Run an ANA with reflex cascade to rule out other autoimmune conditions that may be present aside from UC. Stool cultures can rule out common infections, and a comprehensive stool analysis can give a deeper lens into microbiome diversity, digestion, and potential pathogens present.

Treatment

Dietary Approach

- Eat 1-2 servings of dark berries daily to support small vessels and gut wall healing.
- Eliminate sugar and processed foods.
- Eliminate food intolerances.
- Get 30–50g fiber daily (once an acute flare is past).
- Drink 50–80oz water daily.
- Water fast for two to three days for acute flares (i.e., no food, only water). Food reintroduction needs to be slow, with broths and easily digestible foods initially, like rice, or a flare may worsen and can even get more severe.
- Long-term intermittent fasting may help in maintaining remission (12:12 working to 16:8).

Herbs/Supplements

- Vitamin B Complex – one serving daily
- Magnesium – 300mg one to two times daily
- N-Acetylcysteine – 600mg two to three times daily
- Selenium – 100mcg daily
- Vitamin A – 1500–3000mcg daily
- Vitamin C – 1g two to three times daily
- Vitamin E – 250mg daily
- Vitamin D – 2000–5000IU daily
- Zinc* – 15mg daily
- Iron (if deficient) – 25–50mg daily

INFLAMMATION AND GUT SUPPORT

- Curcumin – 2g twice daily for acute flares. 1g one to two times daily for maintenance.
- High EPA/DHA Fish Oil – 1–2g daily
- Broad Spectrum Probiotic – daily
- Aloe barbadensis leaf pulp/juice – 4oz once or twice daily to heal lesions from flares and for periodic maintenance
- Calendula officinalis tea – 1 tbsp per cup water one to three times daily for acute flares

ACUTE UC FLARE HERBAL TINCTURE FORMULA

Licorice (*Glycyrrhiza glabra*)
Wild Yam (*Dioscorea villosa*)
Fennel (*Foeniculum vulgare*)

Mix 35% Licorice, 35% Wild Yam, 30% Fennel. Take 2–4 droppersful three to four times daily. Stop or decrease once symptoms start to resolve. Monitor blood pressure, as this dose of licorice can cause hypertension as well as potentially cause insomnia. If this happens, blood pressure will return to normal after stopping licorice.

With long-term zinc supplementation, you have to also supplement with 1–3mg/day of copper to avoid zinc-induced copper deficiency.

CHRONIC UC HERBAL TINCTURE FORMULA 2 (IMMUNOMODULATING)

Astragalus *(Astragalus membranaceus)*
Siberian Ginseng *(Eleutherococcus senticosus)*
Devil's Club *(Oplopanax horridus)*
Ashwagandha *(Withania somnifera)*
Licorice *(Glycyrrhiza glabra)*

Mix 25% Astragalus, 25% Siberian Ginseng, 20% Devil's Club, 20% Ashwagandha, 10% Licorice. Take 2–4 droppersful two to three times daily long term as long as it supports remission.

Lifestyle Changes

Sleep is necessary to keep your immune system functioning in a healthy and balanced way. Seven to eight hours a night of uninterrupted sleep is recommended. Pay attention to appropriate quantity but also quality. When sleep is out of balance, the effects are quickly noticeable when it's improved.

Affirmation

I allow any anger, fear, or resentments to transform and leave me with grace.

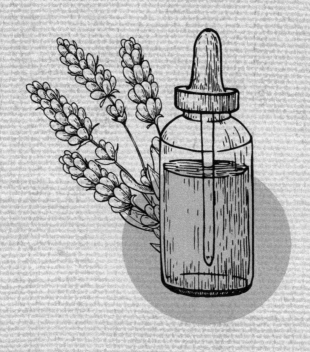

GLOSSARY

ACETYLCHOLINE A neurotransmitter in the brain and elsewhere in the body

ACETYLCHOLINESTERASE An enzyme that breaks down acetylcholine

ADAPTOGEN An herb that doesn't have one effect but a host of effects that give it a generally strengthening and tonifying action. Some actions are immune balancing, increasing blood sugar balance, and modifying the stress response.

ANTI-INFLAMMATORY DIET A diet high in plants, antioxidants, and anti-inflammatory compounds; it is a diet low in pro-inflammatory compounds such as refined sugar, processed foods, and industrially produced seed oils

ANTI-VIRAL A medication, herb, or other compound that has action which prevents and treats viral infections

ANTIOXIDANT A substance that removes oxidative substances from the body

BIOFEEDBACK Using the self, human, electronics, or software as a means to get feedback about the body and physiology in order to increase awareness and ultimately change the physiology and bodily experience

BIOFLAVONOID Antioxidant compounds found in plants that have biological activity; many bioflavonoids are what give fruits and vegetables their dark and bright colors (e.g., quercetin, hesperidin, and isoquercetin)

BPA (BISPHENOL A) An industrial chemical that has been used to make certain plastics and resins since the 1960s that mimics estrogen in the human body

BRONCHODILATION The opening of the bronchi and bronchioles, which are the part of the airway between the trachea and the alveoli where oxygen is exchanged

COMPREHENSIVE NUTRIENT PANEL A blood test that assesses a wide range of nutrients, including B vitamins; a broad range of minerals; many other vitamins like C, E, D, K, A; as well as amino acids; breakdown products; and some include certain heavy metals

COMPREHENSIVE STOOL ANALYSIS A stool test that assesses a variety of factors, such as abundance and diversity of commensal bacteria, presence of pathogens, digestive/absorptive quality, inflammation, and the presence of blood

DECOCT Extraction by heating or boiling; for herbal medicine, a low simmer

DYSBIOSIS, GUT An imbalance in the microbial ecosystem in the intestines; often there is an overgrowth of certain organisms which outcompete with others

ELECTROLYTES Minerals in the body with electric charge such as potassium, magnesium, sodium, etc.

ENDOCANNABINOIDS Neurotransmitters made by the human body that bind to cannabinoid receptors in the brain and elsewhere in the body

EYE MOVEMENT DESENSITIZATION AND REPROCESSING (EMDR) A psychotherapy treatment that was originally designed to alleviate the distress associated with traumatic memories

FOOD ELIMINATION/RE-CHALLENGE DIET A diet meant to eliminate any number of foods in the effort to see symptom improvement from any condition; with symptom improvement, it is known that an eliminated food contributed to symptoms and then a systematic reintroduction every three to four days is done to see which food(s) re-create symptoms

FOOD INTOLERANCE A food that is not tolerated well by the body, resulting in any number of symptoms

GLYCERITE A liquid glycerin extract of an herb

HEART RATE VARIABILITY The variation between heartbeats; it is an indicator of autonomic nervous system balance and tone, which controls the involuntary functions of our body; in general, the greater the variability, the greater the cardiovascular fitness and resilience to stress

HEIDELBERG TEST A test that measures the pH of the stomach and specifically low stomach acid production

HEPATOPROTECTIVE Protective to the liver from oxidation and damage

HIGH-INTENSITY INTERVAL TRAINING (HIIT) An exercise of alternating between bursts of high-intensity exercise and short periods of rest

IMMUNOMODULATION An action of a medication, herb, or other substance that alters the immune system by stimulation, suppression, or balancing; from an herbalism and natural medicine point of view, immunomodulation typically means to balance the immune system

INTERMITTENT FASTING Going 16 or more hours in a 24-hour period without consuming calories; getting all calories in an eight-hour period or less in a 24-hour period

KETO-ADAPTATION The process of the biochemistry of the body shifting to utilize fats for fuel efficiently instead of glucose, which is the typical fuel source

KETOGENIC DIET A low-carb, high-fat diet, which mimics a fasting state metabolically; the body transitions to using fats as the primary fuel source instead of glucose

MOTILITY, GUT The normal contractions and relaxations of the intestines, a.k.a. peristalsis, that moves food and fluids through the digestive tract

NEUROFEEDBACK A type of biofeedback that measures brainwaves and then uses various feedback approaches to enhance and balance their brain functions and utilize underutilized brain pathways

NLR (NEUTROPHIL/LYMPHOCYTE RATIO) An equation of dividing a given two white blood cell numbers for a complete blood count to provide an estimation of systemic inflammation; higher ratio correlates with more inflammation and decreased health outcomes in severe illnesses

NSAID Nonsteroidal anti-inflammatory drugs (e.g., ibuprofen, indomethacin)

PHYTOESTROGEN Plant-derived compounds that mimic estrogen in the body but bind weaker to estrogen receptors than actual estrogen

PROVOKED, HEAVY METAL TESTING The use of chelating agents that heavily bind metals which are then excreted from the body, as means to test heavy metal toxicity

REPLETION, OF NUTRIENTS Replacing nutrients which are deficient

SNP (SINGLE-NUCLEOTIDE POLYMORPHISM) Genetic mutations in a single place that result in an altered function of the protein that the gene encodes for

SEQUELAE A condition which is the consequence of a previous disease or injury

SOMATIC MEDICINE THERAPY A mind-body therapeutic approach that uses body awareness, movement, and bodily experience to process emotion and trauma

STEEP (HERBALISM) To soak in hot water

TINCTURE A liquid alcohol extract of an herb

RESOURCES

Biofeedback and Neurofeedback Resources

Nijmegen Questionnaire hgs.uhb.nhs.uk/wp-content/uploads/Nijmegen_Questionnaire.pdf

Association for Applied Psychophysiology and Biofeedback aapb.org/i4a/pages/index.cfm?pageid=1

International Society for Neurofeedback & Research isnr.org

HeartMath HeartMath.com

Food and Nutrition Resources

My Food Data (lists of foods high in a variety of different vitamins and minerals) MyFoodData.com

Emerson Ecologics (source to buy quality supplements) EmersonEcologics.com

Environmental Working Group ewg.org

Dirty Dozen/Clean Fifteen List ewg.org/foodnews/dirty-dozen.php

Monterey Bay Aquarium Seafood Watch SeafoodWatch.org/seafood-recommendations

Anti-Inflammatory Diet Lifestyle Guide fammed.wisc.edu/files/webfm-uploads/documents/outreach/im/handout_ai_diet_patient.pdf

Food Labeling & Nutrition FDA.gov/food/food-labeling-nutrition

Food Print (guides to various food labels, environmental impacts of different foods, and a lot more) FoodPrint.org

Blue Zones (information gathered from the places on Earth with the longest life expectancies) BlueZones.com

National Institutes of Health (nutrient information) ods.od.nih.gov/factsheets/list-all

Food Allergies and Food Intolerance: The Complete Guide to Their Identification and Treatment by Jonathan Brostoff, MD, and Linda Gamlin

Herbal Medicine Books

Medical Herbalism: The Science and Practice of Herbal Medicine by David Hoffmann, FNIMH, AHG

Herbal Medicine from The Heart of The Earth by Sharol Tilgner, ND

Weiss's Herbal Medicine by Rudolf Fritz Weiss, MD

Herbal Treatment of Children: Western and Ayurvedic Perspectives by Anne McIntyre

Naturally Healthy Babies and Children: A commonsense Guide to Herbal Remedies, Nutrition, and Health by Aviva Jill Romm, MD
Medicinal Plants of the Pacific West by Michael Moore
Practical Wisdom in Natural Healing by Deborah Frances, RN, ND

Homeopathy Resources

The Organon of Medicine by Samuel Hahnemann (Free at HomeopathySchool
.com/the-school/editorial/the-organon)
The Homeopathic Treatment of Children by Paul Herscu, ND
New England School of Homeopathy (a resource for learning and finding a
classical homeopath) Nesh.com

Natural Medicine Historical Books

Nature Doctors: Pioneers in Naturopathic Medicine by Friedhelm Kirchfeld
and Wayde Boyle
Nature Cure by Henry Lindlahr
Vitalism: The History of Herbalism, Homeopathy, and Flower Essences
by Matthew Wood

Naturopathic Doctor Search Resources

American Association of Naturopathic Physicians Naturopathic.org
Association of Accredited Naturopathic Medical Colleges AANMC.org
Institute for Natural Medicine NatureMed.org

Specialty Labs Information

Genova Diagnostics GDX.net
Doctor's Data DoctorsData.com
Diagnostic Solutions Lab DiagnosticSolutionsLab.com
Microbiology Dx (bacterial and mold sinus culture) MicrobiologyDX.com
Great Plains Laboratory GreatPlainsLaboratory.com

Other Resources

Centers for Disease Control and Prevention CDC.gov
JustStand.org JustStand.org
EMDR Institute, Inc. EMDR.com

REFERENCES

Abdul Manap, A.S., S. Vijayabalan, P. Madhavan, Y.Y. Chia, A. Arya, E.H. Wong, F. Rizwan, U. Bindal, and S. Koshy. "*Bacopa monnieri*, a Neuroprotective Lead in Alzheimer Disease: A Review on Its Properties, Mechanisms of Action, and Preclinical and Clinical Studies." *Drug Target Insights* 13 (July 31, 2019). doi: 10.1177/1177392819866412.

Alimujiang, A., A. Wiensch, J. Boss, N.L. Fleischer, A.M. Mondul, K. McLean, B. Mukherjee, and C.L. Pearce. "Association between Life Purpose and Mortality among US Adults Older Than 50 Years." (2019). *JAMA Network Open* 2 no. 5 (2019): e194270. doi.org/10.1001/jamanetworkopen.2019.4270.

Alzheimer's Association. ALZ.org.

American Diabetes Association. Diabetes.org.

American Optometric Association. "Diet and Nutrition" Date accessed July 1, 2020. AOA.org/patients-and-public/caring-for-your-vision/nutrition/nutrition-and-cataracts.

American Society for Gastrointestinal Endoscopy. "Diet and Gastroesphageal Reflux Disease (GERD)." Published 2014. ASGE.org/docs/default-source/about-asge/newsroom/doc-gerd_infographic_final.pdf.

American Thyroid Association. "Graves' Disease." Date accessed July 1, 2020. Thyroid.org/graves-disease.

Anxiety and Depression Association of America. ADAA.org.

Babizhayev, M.A., A.I. Deyev, V.N. Yermakova, Y.A. Semiletov, N.G. Davydova, V.S. Doroshenko, A.V. Zhukotskii, and I.M. Goldman. "Efficacy of N-acetylcarnosine in the treatment of cataracts." *Drugs in R&D* 3, no. 2 (2002): 87–103. doi.org/10.2165/00126839-200203020-00004.

Blue Zones. BlueZones.com.

BMJ Best Practice. "Assessment of Anaemia." Date accessed July 1, 2020. BestPractice.bmj.com/topics/en-gb/93/diagnosis-approach.

Bongiorno, Peter, ND, LAc. "Toxicity and Depression." NDNR. Published March 23, 2012. ndnr.com/mindbody/toxicity-and-depression.

Briden, Lara. *Period Repair Manual: Natural Treatment for Better Hormones and Better Periods*. Scotts Valley, CA: CreateSpace, 2015.

CDC. "Signs and Symptoms of Autism Spectrum Disorders." Last Reviewed August 27, 2019. CDC.gov/ncbddd/autism/signs.html.

Celiac Disease Foundation. Celiac.org.

Centers for Disease Control and Prevention. CDC.gov.

Chemerovski-Glikman, M., M. Mimouni, Y. Dagan, et al. "Rosmarinic Acid Restores Complete Transparency of Sonicated Human Cataract Ex Vivo and Delays Cataract Formation In Vivo." *Scientific Reports* 8, no. 9341 (2018). doi.org/10.1038/s41598-018-27516-9.

Children and Adults with Attention-Deficit/Hyperactivity Disorder (CHADD). CHADD.org.

Chin, K.Y., K.L. Pang, and W.F. Mark-Lee. "A Review on the Effects of Bisphenol A and Its Derivatives on Skeletal Health." *International Journal of Medical Sciences* 15, no. 10 (2018) 1043–50. doi.org/10.7150/ijms.25634.

Choobforoushzadeh, A., Neshat-Doost, H.T., H. Molavi, and M.R. Abedi. "Effect of Neurofeedback Training on Depression and Fatigue in Patients with Multiple Sclerosis. *Applied Psychophysiology and Biofeedback* 40, no. 1 (2015): 1–8. doi.org/10.1007/s10484-014-9267-4.

Christudoss, P., Selvakumar, R., P. Christudoss, J.J. Fleming, and G. Gopalakrishnan. "Zinc Status of Patients with Benign Prostatic Hyperplasia and Prostate Carcinoma. Indian journal of urology: IJU: *Indian Journal of Urology* 27, no. 1 (2011): 14–8. doi: 10.4103/0970-1591.78405.

Conkle, Ann. "Serious Research on Happiness." Association for Psychological Science. Published August 1, 2008. PsychologicalScience.org/observer/serious-research-on-happiness.

Crohn's & Colitis Foundation. "Common Micronutrient Deficiencies in IBD. Educational Resource for Healthcare Providers." Published January 2017. CrohnsColitisFoundation.org/sites/default/files/legacy/science-and-professionals/nutrition-resource-/micronutrient-deficiency-fact.pdf.

Duke, James A. *The Green Pharmacy*: *The Ultimate Compendium of Natural Remedies from the World's Foremost Authority on Healing Herbs*. Pennsylvania: Rodale Press, 1997.

Eligio, P., Delia, R., and G. Valeria. "EBV Chronic Infections." *Mediterranean Journal of Hematology and Infectious Diseases* 2, no. 1 (2010): e2010022. doi.org/10.4084/MJHID.2010.022.

EMDR Institute, Inc. EMDR.com.

Gaby, Alan R., MD. *Nutritional Medicine*. New Hampshire: Fritz Perlberg Publishing, 2011.

Güraǧaç, A., and Z. Demirer. "The Neutrophil-to-Lymphocyte Ratio in Clinical Practice." *Canadian Urological Association Journal* 10 no. 3–4 (2016): 141. doi: 10.5489/cuaj.3587.

Hammond, D. Corydon. "What is Neurofeedback: An Update." *Journal of Neurotherapy* 15, no. 4, (2011): 305–36, doi: 10.1080/10874208.2011.623090.

Hoffmann, David. *Medical Herbalism: The Science and Practice of Herbal Medicine*. Vermont: Healing Arts Press, 2003.

International OCD Foundation. "Exposure and Response Prevention." Date accessed July 1, 2020. iocdf.org/about-ocd/ocd-treatment/erp.

JustStand.org. JustStand.org.

Koopmans, T.A., J.M. Geleijnse, F.G. Zitman, and E.J. Giltay. "Effects of Happiness on All-Cause Mortality during 15 years of Follow-up: The Arnhem Elderly Study. *Journal of Happiness Studies: An Interdisciplinary Forum on Subjective Well-Being* 11, no. 1 (2010): 113–24. doi.org/10.1007/s10902-008-9127-0.

Ku, P.W., A. Steptoe, Y. Liao, M.C. Hsueh, and L.J. Chen. "A Cut-off of Daily Sedentary Time and All-Cause Mortality in Adults: a Meta-Regression Analysis Involving More Than 1 Million Participants." *BMC Medicine* 16, no. 1 (2018): 74. doi.org/10.1186/s12916-018-1062-2.

Lehmann, I., U. Sack, and J. Lehmann. "Metal Ions Affecting the Immune System." *Metal Ions in Life Sciences* 8 (2011): 157–85.

Luijmes, Robin, Sjaak Poouwels, and Jacko Boonman. "The Effectiveness of Neurofeedback on Cognitive Functioning in Patients with Alzheimer's Disease: Preliminary Results." *Clinical Neurophysiology* 46, no. 3 (2016): 179–87. doi.org/10.1016/j.neucli.2016.05.069.

Mayo Clinic. "Uterine Fibroids." Date accessed July 1, 2020. MayoClinic.org/diseasesconditions/uterine-fibroids/symptoms-causes/syc-20354288.

Mecdad, A.A., M.H. Ahmed, M.E. ElHalwagy, and M.M. Afify. "A Study on Oxidative Stress Biomarkers and Immunomodulatory Effects of Pesticides in Pesticide-Sprayers." *Egyptian Journal of Forensic Sciences* 1, no. 2 (2011) 93–8. doi.org/10.1016/j.ejfs.2011.04.012.

Medscape. emedicine.medscape.com.

Merck Manual. MerckManuals.com/professional.

Mind Tools. "SMART Goals: How To Make Your Goals Achievable." Date accessed July 1, 2020. MindTools.com/pages/article/smart-goals.htm.

Montgomery E. B., Jr. "Heavy Metals and the Etiology of Parkinson's Disease and Other Movement Disorders." *Toxicology* 97, no. 1–3 (March 31, 1995): 3–9. doi: 10.1016/0300-483x(94)02962-t.

Mount Sinai. "Fibroocystic Breast Disease." Last Reviewed 10/30/2018. MountSinai.org/health-library/diseases-conditions/fibrocystic-breast-disease.

Mullington, J.M., N.S. Simpson, H.K. Meier-Ewert and M. Haack. "Sleep Loss and Inflammation." *Best Practice & Research. Clinical Endocrinology & Metabolism* 24, no. 5 (October 2010): 775–84. doi.org/10.1016/j.beem.2010.08.014.

National Autism Association. NationalAutismAssociation.org.

National Health Service. "Fibromyalgia." Last Reviewed 2/20/2019. NHS.uk/conditions/fibromyalgia.

National Institute of Diabetes and Digestive and Kidney Diseases. "Symptoms and Causes of Crohn's Disease." Last updated September 2017. niddk.nih.gov/health-information/digestive-diseases/crohns-disease/symptoms-causes.

National Institutes of Health, Office of Dietary Supplements. "Dietary Supplement Fact Sheets." ods.od.nih.gov/factsheets/list-all.

National Institutes of Mental Health. "Attention-Deficit/Hyperactivity Disorder (ADHD): The Basics." Revised 2016. nimh.nih.gov/health/publications/attention-deficit-hyperactivity-disorder-adhd-the-basics/index.shtml.

National Organization for Rare Disorders. "Heavy Metal Poisoning." 2006. RareDiseases.org/rare-diseases/heavy-metal-poisoning.

Niemeyer, K., Bell, I.R., and M. Koithan. "Traditional Knowledge of Western Herbal Medicine and Complex Systems Science." *Journal of Herbal Medicine* 3 no. 3 (September 2013): 112–19. doi.org/10.1016/j.hermed.2013.03.001.

Patel, Sheila, MD. "Ask Dr. Sheila: What is Ayurveda?" The Chopra Center. Last updated August 7, 2020. Chopra.com/articles/what-is-ayurveda.

Pizzorno J. "Is the Diabetes Epidemic Primarily Due to Toxins?" *Integrative Medicine* 15, no. 4 (2016): 8–17.

Sandström, B. "Diagnosis of Zinc Deficiency and Excess in Individuals and Populations." *Food and Nutrition Bulletin* 22, no. 2 (2001): 133–37. doi.org/10.1177/156482650102200203.

Siegmann, E.M., H. Müller, C. Luecke, A. Philipsen, J. Kornhuber, and T.W. Gromer. "Association of Depression and Anxiety Disorders with Autoimmune Thyroiditis: A Systematic Review and Meta-analysis." *JAMA Psychiatry* 75, no. 6 (2018): 577–84. doi.org/10.1001/jamapsychiatry.2018.0190.

Singh, R., R.C. Turner, L. Nguyen, K. Motwani, M. Swatek, B.P. Lucke-Wold, and R. Qaiser. "Pediatric Traumatic Brain Injury and Autism: Elucidating Shared Mechanisms." *Behavioural Neurology* (2016) doi.org/10.1155 /2016/8781725.

Steptoe, Andrew. "Happiness and Health." *Annual Review of Public Health* 40 (April 2019): 339–359. doi.org/10.1146/annurev-publhealth-040218-044150.

Thor, J.A., N.H. Mohamed Hanapi, H. Halil, and A. Suhaimi. "Perineural Injection Therapy in the Management of Complex Regional Pain Syndrome: A Sweet Solution to Pain." *Pain Medicine* 18, no. 10 (October 2017): 2041–45. doi.org/10.1093/pm/pnx063.

Tilgner, Sharol Marie. *Herbal Medicine from the Heart of the Earth*. Pleasant Hill, OR: Wise Acres, LLC, 2009.

Tradition Chinese Medicine World Foundation. "What is TCM?" Date accessed July 1, 2020. TCMWorld. org. https://www.tcmworld.org/what-is-tcm

Wilkins, T., K. Jarvis, and J. Patel. "Diagnosis and Management of Crohn's Disease." *American Family Physician* 84, no. 12 (December 2011): 1365–75.

Wilt, T., A. Ishani, R. MacDonald, G. Stark, C. Mulrow, and J. Lau. "Beta-sitosterols for Benign Prostatic Hyperplasia. *The Cochrane Database of Systematic Reviews* 2 (2000): CD001043. doi.org/10.1002/ 14651858.CD001043.

Włodarek D. "Role of Ketogenic Diets in Neurodegenerative Diseases (Alzheimer's Disease and Parkinson's Disease)." *Nutrients* 11, no. 1 (2019): 169 doi.org/10.3390/nu11010169.

Wolraich, M L., J.F. Hagan, Jr., C. Allan, E. Chan, D. Davison, M. Earls, S.W. Evans, S.K. Flinn, T. Froehlich, J. Frost, J.R. Holbrook, J. R., et. al. "Clinical Practice Guideline for the Diagnosis, Evaluation, and Treatment of Attention-Deficit/Hyperactivity Disorder in Children and Adolescents." *Pediatrics* 144, no. 4 (2019): e20192528. doi.org/10.1542/peds.2019-2528.

Worley S. L. "The Extraordinary Importance of Sleep: The Detrimental Effects of Inadequate Sleep on Health and Public Safety Drive an Explosion of Sleep Research." *P & T* 43, no. 12 (2018): 758–63.

Yarnell, Eric. *Natural Approach to Gastroenterology. 2nd ed.* Washington: Healing Mountain Publishing, 2010.

INDEX

V

Valerian*, 52
vitamin B complex, 32
vitamin C, 42, 55

W

wellness
 goals, 24, 25–27
 plan for, 25, 28
Western Herbalism (WH), 6, 7

*See important information.

Y

yoga, 5, 17, 75, 111, 127, 161

Z

Zinc
 supplement information*, 59, 63, 66,
  70, 130, 139, 175, 178, 182

ACKNOWLEDGMENTS

This book would not have come to fruition if not for the support of my wife, Sarah Sue. She made the space for me to spend long hours at the office as well as many weekends researching and writing. She made me food to keep my brain and body going and gave me peace of mind knowing that Leo had an amazing mother taking care of him. She truly has supported my mind, body, and spirit in this process.

I'm grateful for my time in the army and the doctors and nurses who mentored me. I had the incredible opportunity as a 19- and 20-year-old to assist in surgery, start hundreds of IVs, suture children's lacerations, perform arterial blood gases, and so much more. I would not have gone down this path if not for this early experience and the inspiration those people provided me.

My time in naturopathic medical school introduced me to amazing teachers, doctors, and healers, some of whom have become close friends. Greg Yasuda, ND, and Brad Lichtenstein, ND, were the first doctors that I realized were also healers and demonstrated to me the healthy masculine. They lit a fire in me for the healing power of nature, the art of practicing medicine, and the sacredness of the doctor-patient relationship. Pamela Snider, ND, was my first teacher of the philosophy of naturopathic medicine. She articulated it in a way that I was able to understand how to apply it as an effective guide for my treatments. I have Durr Elmore, ND, DC; Paul Herscu, ND; and Amy Rothenburg, ND; to thank for enlightening me to the field of homeopathy, its beauty, and its power. Lastly, of my medicine teachers, I have Bruce Milliman, ND, to thank. Our discussions and my time working with him while a student taught me how to use the right tools for the job at the right time, whether natural or pharmaceutical, in order to keep the patient safe and get them well quickly.

Finally, I give thanks for the gift of prayer. Thank you, Creator, for hearing my prayers and bringing me into the world with the ability to see the path forward, in order to find healing for those who have long been suffering.

ABOUT THE AUTHOR

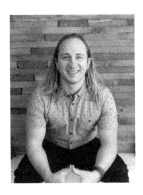

DR. BLAKE MYERS is a widely respected naturopathic physician, author, and educator of natural medicine. Based out of Bellingham, Washington, he is the owner and founder of Chiron Healing Arts, a naturopathic and homeopathic clinic with a special interest in treating patients with complex chronic illness and chronic pain. Dr. Myers was a medic in the US Army. He has a bachelor of science in biology from Iowa State University of Science and Technology and earned his doctor of naturopathic medicine degree from Bastyr University. Starting his career in primary care, Dr. Myers began seeing patients with longstanding health problems of many years, often decades, improving with his unique treatment approach. He worked in a specialty addiction medicine clinic for three years, where he realized his full potential to help transform the lives of people with chronic illness and chronic pain. Dr. Myers has served as the vice president of the Naturopathic Academy of Primary Care Physicians (NAPCP) and has served as a mentoring physician in Seattle, Washington, at the Integrative Care Outreach (ICO), a community-based integrative medicine organization serving homeless and extreme low-income populations.

Instagram @Dr._Blake
DrBlakeMyers.com

CPSIA information can be obtained
at www.ICGtesting.com
Printed in the USA
JSHW022135061120
9315JS00003B/3

9 781647 395216